"Share this engaging book with an anxious child and give them  of freedom from anxiety."

> —**Elizabeth DuPont Spencer, LCSW-C**, therapist, author ~~...~~ Anxiety
> *Cure for Kids*, and cofounder of Anxiety Training

"The book is such a fun and engaging way to help your child learn the life-changing principles of overcoming anxiety, that even the most scared kid will find it engaging. Elementary-aged children will discover easy, relatable ways to understand, challenge, and master their fears using the very best strategies science has to offer. It is sure to become a favorite amongst parents and therapists!"

> —**Karen Lynn Cassiday, PhD**, past president of the Anxiety and Depression
> Association of America; owner of the Anxiety Treatment Center of Greater
> Chicago; and author of books helping parents, children, and adults
> overcome anxiety

"*The Anxiety Busting Workbook for Kids* is a fabulous cognitive behavioral therapy (CBT) workbook for kids with anxiety. It's engaging and jam-packed with evidence-based strategies to help kids overcome fears—and delivered in a fun, creative, and adorable format. This will be a fast favorite!"

> —**Rachel Busman, PsyD, ABPP**, senior director of the Child and Adolescent
> Anxiety Program at Cognitive and Behavioral Consultants

"This book is a great resource for the clinician working with anxious children or tweens! Using a combination of engaging graphics and storytelling, these authors guide the youth through understanding, engaging, and taming their anxieties, fears, and worries. Whether it's used in an individual, group, or family setting, this book will help clinicians help kids and those who love them deal with anxiety."

> —**Tony L. Sheppard, PsyD, CGP, ABPP, AGPA-F**, founder and director of
> Groupworks Psychological Services, and coauthor of *Group Psychotherapy
> with Children*

"The Anxiety Busting Workbook for Kids is such a treasure! Step by step, this workbook takes parents and kids through the process of understanding anxiety and how to respond so that kids can get back to enjoying their lives without fearing anxiety. The creative activities help children learn evidence-based practices while having fun and earning rewards. Any child would benefit from learning these skills."

> **—Kimberly Morrow, LCSW**, anxiety therapist, cofounder of Anxiety Training, and author of *Face It and Feel It*

"The Anxiety Busting Workbook for Kids provides an incredibly creative approach for helping kids learn to identify and overcome their fears. It does a wonderful job of incorporating complex CBT strategies in a very user-friendly manner for children. I would highly recommend this book for children with anxiety."

> **—Brian J. Schmaus**, clinical psychologist at the Anxiety Treatment Center of Greater Chicago in Deerfield, IL

The Anxiety Busting Workbook for Kids

Fun CBT Activities to Squash Your Fears & Worries

Debra Kissen, PhD
Meena Dugatkin, PsyD
Grace Cusack, LPC

Instant Help Books
An Imprint of New Harbinger Publications, Inc.

Publisher's Note

INSTANT HELP, the Clock Logo, and NEW HARBINGER are trademarks of New Harbinger Publications, Inc.

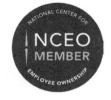

Distributed in Canada by Raincoast Books

Cover design by Sara Christian

Interior book design by Tom Comitta

Acquired by Jennye Garibaldi

Edited by Gretel Hakanson

Printed in the United States of America

26   25   24

10   9   8   7   6   5   4   3   2   1   First Printing

This book is dedicated to you amazing kids,
together with your parents and loved ones,
who bravely faced and conquered your worries
and fears. Your courage and adventurous spirit
inspired us to write this book. We learned and
grew together by trying out creative exercises to
make the journey of moving through and past
anxiety fun and exciting. Thank you for being
our incredible teachers and guides!

Contents

Foreword   vi

A Note to Kids   viii

A Note to Parents   x

ACTIVITY 1   Your Fear Busting Adventure   2

ACTIVITY 2   Build-a-Bank Workshop   9

ACTIVITY 3   Brave Prize Wish List   15

ACTIVITY 4   Guard Dog Within   18

ACTIVITY 5   Bark Translator   23

ACTIVITY 6   What Breed Is Your Guard Dog?   29

ACTIVITY 7   How to Train Your Guard Dog   43

ACTIVITY 8   Scary Feeling IScream Shop   49

ACTIVITY 9   Your Body on Fear   56

ACTIVITY 10   Breathing Pop It   65

ACTIVITY 11   Thought-Feeling-Action Loopty-Loop   69

ACTIVITY 12   Your Dream Pizza   75

ACTIVITY 13   Focus Pocus   79

ACTIVITY 14   Hoo Hoo? Your Wise Owl, That's Who!   82

ACTIVITY 15   Healthy Competition   93

ACTIVITY 16 Mindfulness Express Train 97

ACTIVITY 17 Mindful Coloring 101

ACTIVITY 18 Scary Pie Bake-Off 105

ACTIVITY 19 From "Wow" to "Whatever" 111

ACTIVITY 20 Fear Transformer 116

ACTIVITY 21 Rolling in Your Fears 120

ACTIVITY 22 Scary Land 123

ACTIVITY 23 The Get It Wrong Game 129

ACTIVITY 24 Best in Show 134

ACTIVITY 25 BraveWare 140

Celebration Station! 148

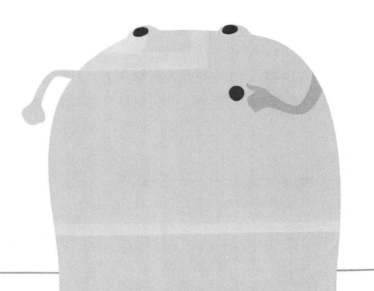

Foreword

Anxiety problems in children (as well as adults) have never been more prevalent. Rates of childhood anxiety disorders seem to rise steadily, and even children and teens who are not experiencing a clinical level of anxiety that would warrant formal diagnosis are facing more and more anxiety-related struggles in their daily lives. The reasons for why anxiety has been on the rise are complex and largely unknown. What is known is that it is possible to reduce anxiety and to limit its impact on a child's life. If you are a young person coping with anxiety in your life, or if you have a young person who is coping with anxiety in their life, you are holding the right book—you've "come to the right place."

Decades of research and clinical experience have led to an ever-richer understanding of tools that can be used to overcome anxiety in young people. These tools generally have their roots in cognitive, behavioral, and physiological science and their application in cognitive-behavioral therapy, or CBT. The principles behind these tools are surprisingly simple and easy to grasp. In fact, most of them are already known, even to children. For example, it is well-known that repetition dulls emotional impact. This psychological principle is common to so much lived experience that it is generally taken for granted. (The first sunny day after a long gray winter tends to make people happy. The tenth sunny day in a row, not as much.) Tools for overcoming anxiety leverage this and other principles that are generally also simple, straightforward, and familiar. Yet while the principles may be simple and straightforward, actually learning to cope with anxiety is not. As any experienced clinician can attest, the tricky part in helping a person to overcome anxiety is not figuring out the tools to use – it is presenting those tools in such a way that the person will actually use them.

That is precisely where I believe this book will excel. The creativity that the authors have infused into the activities described throughout the book and their own infectious enthusiasm communicated on page after page will make it easy for children to try out these tools. The sense of fun and adventure that suffuses the workbook makes working through it a bit like visiting the office of a particularly gifted child psychologist. One who can draw a child in, partner with them on a grand adventure, and lead them through the work of therapy without it feeling like work at all.

This book will also provide you, the parent, with the words for presenting the tools to your child and with suggestions for how you and your child can work together. Using these words and following the suggestions can help you to avoid some nasty pitfalls. Even a well-intentioned parent can fall into these traps, such as prodding a child too forcefully to use a tool, so that the result is resentment instead of motivation. With twenty-five different activities work through, if one activity is not a good fit for your particular child or for this particular moment, there will be another to try.

Working through the activities in the book will require some investment of time and energy. I can think of no better use of a parent's time than helping their child to learn to live better with anxiety. If your child learns to manage their anxiety better, to fear it less, to face it rather than run from it, to take control of it rather than being controlled by it, to communicate and express it rather than trying to always repress it, to find the humor in it rather than only the grim, perhaps even to embrace it rather than trying to erase it…if your child learns even one of these things, your investment of time and energy will pay off many times over. The impact of anxiety on a child's life can be extensive. The impact of learning to live better with anxiety is equally far-reaching.

—ELI R. LEBOWITZ, PHD

A Note to Kids

We all get scared and worried sometimes, and guess what? This is actually a really good thing! Feeling afraid is like having a super-duper guard dog inside you, always ready to keep you safe and sound.

Imagine this: You're getting ready to leave for school, and then you start having an uncomfortable worried feeling. This is your guard dog coming to your rescue, saying, "Hold up! Something important needs your attention!" You then realize you forgot to put your homework in your backpack and it's still on the kitchen counter where you were working on it last night.

But sometimes feeling scared and worried is not as helpful. These are the moments when you feel all the discomfort of fear without any of the benefits of safety. In these moments, there is nothing bad or dangerous happening and you do not need protection.

Imagine this: You and your family are starving and decide to make it a pizza night. Soon, a friendly pizza delivery person is at your door, ready to hand you and your hungry family a yummy, sizzling treat. And there is your guard dog, barking loudly at the helpful deliverer of your scrumptious meal. In moments like this, your guard dog is making your life more difficult and less fun.

This book is here to help you with these kinds of false-alarm moments, the ones when your guard dog believes there is danger, but in reality you are safe and sound (and just looking to sit back, relax, and enjoy some yummy pizza!).

You and your chosen adult are about to embark on a brave adventure. Together you will train your guard dog to bark less when the coast is clear and there are no challenges to manage. Soon your guard dog will be sounding the "danger alarm" less often and snuggling up for some well-deserved rest and relaxation more often.

Learning new skills to worry less and have more fun is going to be hard but important work. And just like your parents or anyone else, you are going to get "paid" for your efforts with Brave Points and prizes after you complete the activities throughout this book (more on this in Activities 2 and 3).

We are so excited for you to soon experience how fabulous it feels to be the proud owner of a well-trained guard dog. Your world will grow bigger, and your fears will shrink to a smidgen of their original size.

And with these words, we wish you a silly, messy, fun-packed fear busting adventure!

A Note to Parents

The experience of anxiety can be terrifying, no matter what age you are. But for children, it can be all the more bewildering because they do not yet have the language or advanced cognitive capabilities to describe or make sense of what is unfolding in their mind and body when operating on fear and anxiety. And for the parents of a child experiencing frequent, life-interfering anxiety symptoms, it can be heartbreaking to watch their child's world grow smaller and smaller, as they give up more and more of their life to avoid contact with this nameless, faceless enemy.

The good news is that anxiety disorders in children are the most treatable class of mental health conditions. This book offers a compilation of best-in-class, evidence-based tools and techniques to help your child play their way past fear, anxiety, and worry. Moving past anxiety need not feel like work for your child. In fact, laughing and getting silly with anxiety is the most powerful fear-extinguishing agent around. Anxiety sends the message, "This is very serious! Do not let your guard down. You must remain on high alert." By responding to anxiety with joy and levity, anxiety shrinks to a shadow of its former self.

You play a critical role as a changemaker in helping your child develop a new relationship with their fears, worries, and anxiety. You (or another loved one) will be serving as their adult partner throughout this book. An adult partner's participation in this brave adventure is critical because healthy coping behaviors must be reinforced to become automatic and easily accessible for day-to-day use. For all of us, it is much easier to revert to our old ways, even if they are less effective, than to do something new and effortful. For your child to obtain long-lasting results, they need an adult partner to come along with them on this anxiety busting adventure.

One important way you will be helping your child worry less and have more fun is by providing them with Brave Points as they complete the anxiety squashing exercises throughout this workbook. We all deserve to get rewarded for our hard work, and your child will most certainly be working hard as they learn to think and behave in new and more adaptive ways. By the time your child completes this book, they will have the opportunity to earn 25 Brave Points to use for a special prize of their choosing. The Brave Points and prize they earn will forever serve as a reminder that you believe in them and are so proud of the effort they are putting into squashing their fears and worries.

We do understand how busy and jam-packed a parent's life can be with so many critical and competing demands for your time and attention. So here is our plug for you to openly and actively assist your child in working their way through this activity book: the investment of time and energy you make in this anxiety squashing adventure has the potential to transform not only your child's life but yours as well. Each activity will have a section for your child to complete as well as a section for them to complete with you. By opening up to the work of learning to relate to your fears and worries in a new and more adaptive manner, you too will obtain enhanced anxiety management skills.

And with these words, we wish you a silly, messy, fun-packed fear busting adventure!

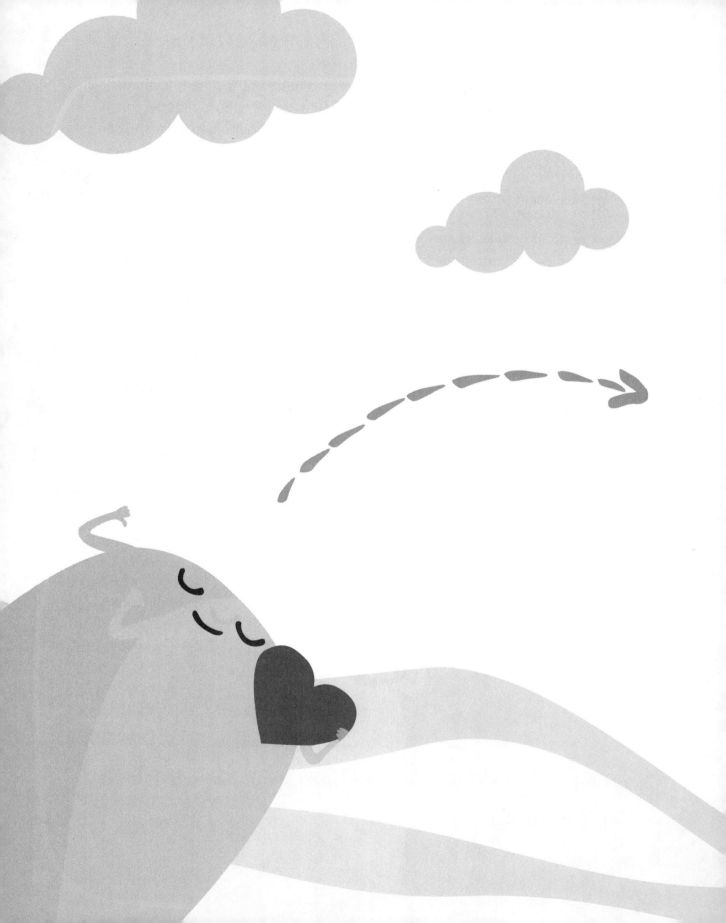

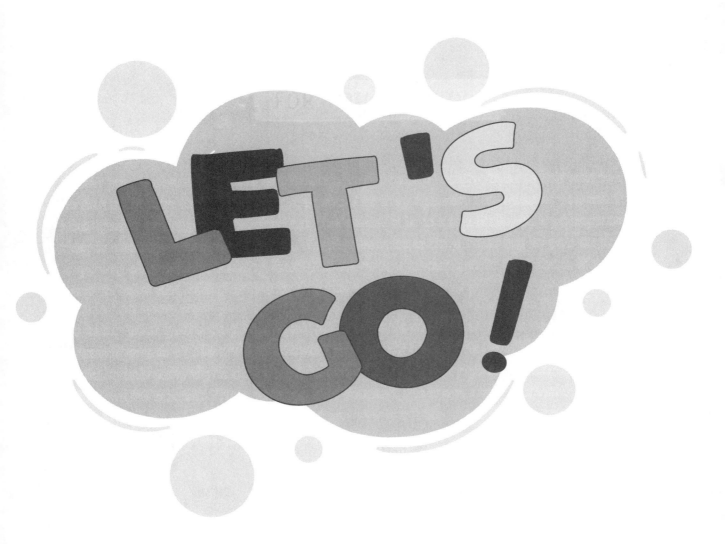

Your Fear Busting Adventure

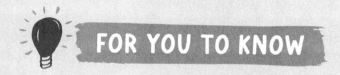

FOR YOU TO KNOW

This book is here to help you learn how to play your way past fears and worries. Yep, you read that right! You can have *fun* while shrinking your fears and worries. Throughout this book, you will have the chance to do all sorts of fun, silly, fear busting challenges and earn plenty of points and prizes along the way.

1. YOUR FEAR BUSTING ADVENTURE

2. BUILD-A-BANK WORKSHOP

START HERE

4. GUARD DOG WITHIN

3. BRAVE PRIZE WISH LIST

5. BARK TRANSLATOR

6. WHAT BREED IS YOUR GUARD DOG?

7. HOW TO TRAIN YOUR GUARD DOG

8. SCARY FEELING ISCREAM SHOP

9. YOUR BODY
ON FEAR

10. BREATHING
POP IT

11. THOUGHT-FEELING-
ACTION LOOPTY-LOOP

13. FOCUS
POCUS

14. HOO HOO?
YOUR WISE OWL,
THAT'S WHO!

12. YOUR
DREAM PIZZA

15. HEALTHY
COMPETITION

16. MINDFULNESS
EXPRESS TRAIN

18. SCARY PIE
BAKE-OFF

17. MINDFUL
COLORING

19. FROM "WOW"
TO "WHATEVER"

20. FEAR
TRANSFORMER

22. SCARY
LAND

21. ROLLING IN
YOUR FEARS

23. THE GET IT
WRONG GAME

25. BRAVEWARE

26. CELEBRATION STATION!

24. BEST
IN SHOW

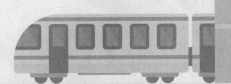

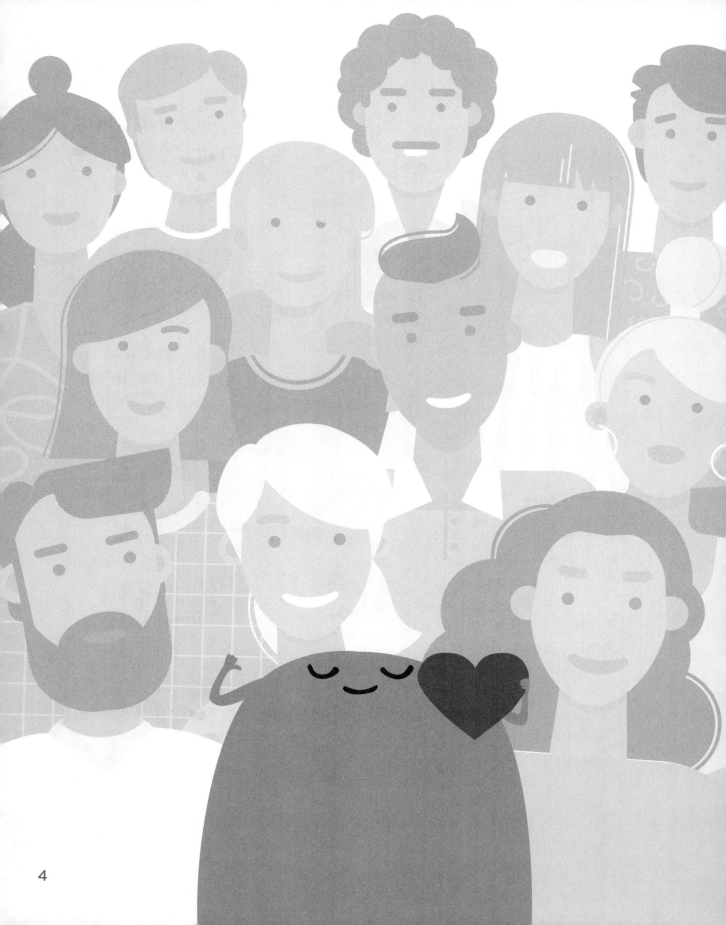

Guess what? You're not the only one who is going to have a fear busting adventure. You get to choose an adult partner to go on this journey with you.

All sorts of people can be your adult partner. Who can you ask?

You can ask:

- an older sibling

- a parent

- other family members (including an aunt, uncle, or grandparent)

- a teacher

- a school counselor

- a therapist

- a coach

- any adult in your life you trust and enjoy spending time with.

The good news is that there are so many people who care about you, believe in you, and would love to join you on this anxiety squashing adventure.

FOR YOU TO DO ⭐

It is time to pick your adult partner.

- Think of someone you trust.

- Think of someone you can count on to be there for you.

- Think of someone who has their own worries, who would also benefit from going on this fear busting adventure.

Who will you ask to be your adult partner?

_____

Name two reasons you picked this person to be your adult partner:

1. _____

2. _____

Now it is time to officially invite your selected adult to join you on this fear squashing adventure.

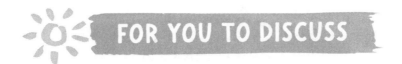
Talk to your adult partner about:

- Why you chose them to join you on this adventure.

- One thing you are hoping to get out of this anxiety squashing adventure and ask them what they are hoping to get out of it.

- One thing about this fear busting adventure that makes you worried and ask them to tell you one thing that worries them.

- What your life would be like if you felt less scared and anxious and ask them to describe the same to you.

- Have them complete the Adult Partner Contract form below.

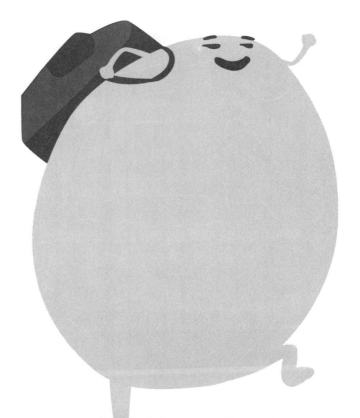

ADULT PARTNER CONTRACT

I _____ (ADULT PARTNER NAME) am available to join

_____ (YOUR NAME) on this important mission. I promise

to be there each step of the way and to encourage _____

(YOUR NAME) to try all of the fear busting activities throughout this book. I promise

to try all of the activities myself as well, as I too would love to worry less and have

more fun. I also promise to help keep track of all the Brave Points earned and will

provide _____ (YOUR NAME) with the prizes earned

based on the reward system we create together.

_____

YOUR SIGNATURE

_____

YOUR ADULT PARTNER'S SIGNATURE

ACTIVITY 2

Build-a-Bank Workshop

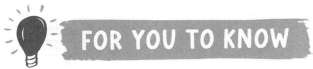

FOR YOU TO KNOW

The true "prize" for completing the activities throughout this book will be a stronger, more powerful you, living a life with smaller fears and more fun!

But it is going to take a bit of practice thinking and acting in new ways. Your fears and worries will shrink to teeny tiny versions of their former selves. Then you will notice how much better you are feeling.

In the meantime, you deserve to earn rewards along the way, as you put in the hard, important work of strengthening your fear busting mental muscles. In fact, everyone deserves rewards to keep them motivated as they complete challenging but important life tasks. Your parents deserve to get paid for the effort they put into their jobs, and you deserve to be rewarded for all the hard work you are going to do in this fear busting adventure.

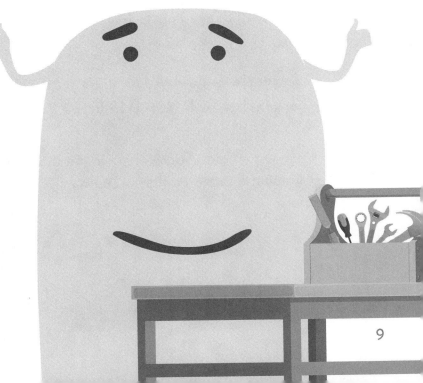

As you complete each fear busting activity throughout this book, you will earn a Brave Point. And when you complete this book, you will have earned a total of 25 Brave Points.

FOR YOU TO DO

1. Gather supplies: scissors, 1 plastic bag, 1 clean glass jar or plastic container, art supplies, and a copy of the 25 Brave Points sheet.

2. Color and decorate the 25 Brave Points.

3. Follow the lines to cut the Brave Points sheet into 25 separate squares.

4. Label plastic bag "Brave Points to Be Earned."

5. Place all Brave Points in this bag.

6. Decorate and label the glass jar or plastic container: "My Brave Points."

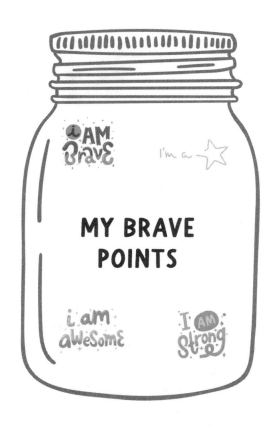

You have just created your very own (fabulous) Brave Points Bank where you will store all the Brave Points you earn as you move through this fear busting adventure.

I am brave	brave	I'm a ⭐	• I AM • STRONG	I AM Strong
i AM BRAVE	BE BRAVE	BE BRAVE	Brave	Be Brave
brave	BE BRAVE	YOU ARE BRAVE	BE BRAVE	Brave
I DID IT!	GO ME!	I am BRAVE	I AM STRONG	PROUD to be ME!
I believe in me	i am awesome	Be Brave	yay	i AM BRAVE

11

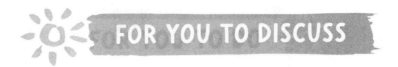

Ask your adult partner:

- Would you continue to work at your job if you no longer got paid?

- How does receiving a paycheck help you to keep showing up for work, especially on days when you are feeling tired and would much rather stay in bed, under your cozy covers?

- Do you think I deserve rewards for the hard, important work of shrinking my fears and worries?

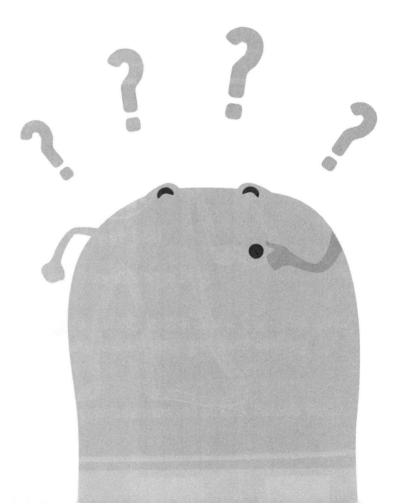

CONGRATULATIONS!

You just earned a 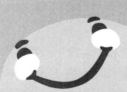. Plus, give yourself a Brave Point for completing Activity 1.

So you have already earned two Brave Points. Great work!

★ Take two Brave Point coupons from the storage bag.

★ On the back of each Brave Point, write down (or have your adult partner write down) one thing you learned by completing the activity.

★ Place the Brave Point in your supercool Brave Points Bank.

ACTIVITY 3

Brave Prize Wish List

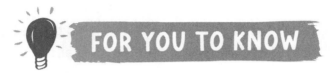

FOR YOU TO KNOW

It's time to talk PRIZES! You and your adult partner need to decide what awesome prizes you can earn in exchange for your Brave Points.

For example, a supercool kid who squashed her worries decided to use her Brave Points to earn the prizes below.

One brave point equals a special activity, such as having friends over for a sleepover, movie night, or going to a trampoline park.

5 points equals an Amazon or Target gift card.

10 points equals a new video game.

25 points equals a family adventure weekend.

Now it is your turn. Talk with your adult partner and together come up with a list of possible rewards. And keep in mind, this does not have to be your final list of prizes. These are just some ideas of prizes and rewards you may want to earn. You can change your mind at any time, so you don't have to come up with the perfect list. The point of this activity is just to get you thinking about the fun prizes you can earn as you make your way through this fear busting adventure. Write down your ideas below.

MY BRAVE PRIZES WISH LIST

(1 Point) [   ]

(5 Points) [   ]

(10 Points) [   ]

(20 Points) [   ]

(25 Points) [   ]

☀ FOR YOU TO DISCUSS

Take turns answering these questions with your adult partner. After hearing each other's responses, take a moment to compliment each other for bravely discussing this important topic.

- How would you want to reward yourself for the hard but important work of squashing your fears?

- If you could earn 25 Brave Points, what prize would you choose for yourself?

- Can you give yourself this prize when we both finish this book?

By completing this activity, you have earned a

Great job!

★ **Take a Brave Point from the storage bag.**

★ **On the back of the Brave Point, write down (or have your adult partner write down) one thing you learned by completing the activity.**

★ **Place the Brave Point in your supercool Brave Points Bank.**

ACTIVITY 4

Guard Dog Within

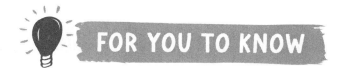

Have you ever felt afraid or worried about something even though there was nothing obviously bad or scary happening around you?

It may seem like your brain is just trying to mess with you by making you feel stressed and anxious when there is nothing actually wrong. But, believe it or not, your brain is actually trying to protect you from what it mistakenly thinks is a dangerous situation.

Your brain is incredibly powerful. It has different parts that play important roles and work together to help you do all the important things you need to do, like walking, talking, and eating. In this book, you're going to learn about two important parts of your brain: your Feeling Brain and your Thinking Brain.

Your Feeling Brain is really fast and acts quickly based on its first impression of what's happening. It's like a guard dog that barks at strangers without thinking about whether it's safe or dangerous.

Just like a real-life guard dog, your guard dog (in other words, your Feeling Brain) is quick to "bark" and think there is danger even when there is nothing actually wrong.

A guard dog might bark at the mailman when they walk by your house to deliver your mail. Similarly, your guard dog may bark to warn you of danger when you are at a friend's birthday party. These are false alarms.

Imagine a strange tree with curvy branches. Your guard dog could be quick to think, *Oh no!! Snake!!*

A few moments later, your Thinking Brain may look more carefully at the tree and then let you know, "That was just a false alarm. There is no snake in the tree. That was just a strange curvy branch!"

In this situation, it makes sense for your guard dog to first think, *Danger!* and then look for clues to find out if this tree would be safe to climb. After all, who wants to climb a snakey tree? Ick!!

So, there are times when you want your guard dog to be very careful and warn you of danger, even if that means dealing with a loud, uncomfortable false alarm.

Because we don't live outside anymore, we will not bump into too many snakes on a normal day (hopefully!). But there will be times our guard dog will think safe situations are dangerous.

And getting so many false-alarm messages from your guard dog can make you feel stressed out, anxious, and super uncomfortable.

The good news is that your guard dog is trainable. This activity book will help you train your guard dog to get better at telling the difference between true danger and when you are safe and sound. And once your guard dog learns it is safe enough to stop barking, you will feel less scared and uncomfortable in your body. Most importantly, you will be able to get back to doing the things you love most!

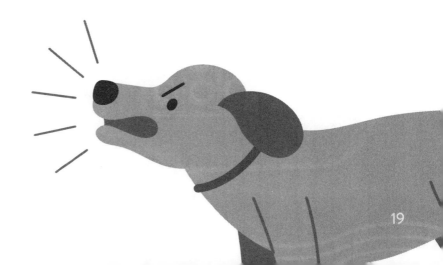

1. Place an X on the moments when a guard dog is barking about something that isn't actually a danger.

2. Place a ✓ on the moments when it is a good idea for a guard dog to bark and warn of danger.

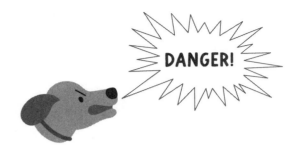

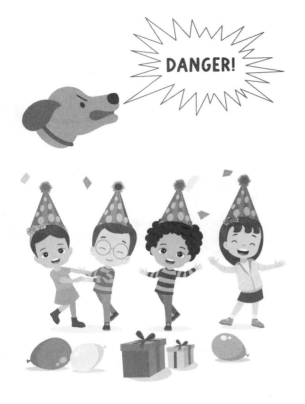

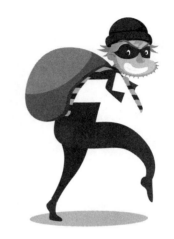

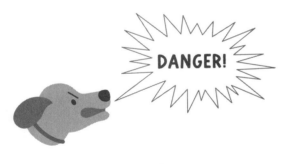

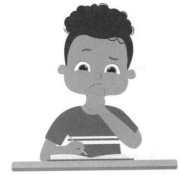

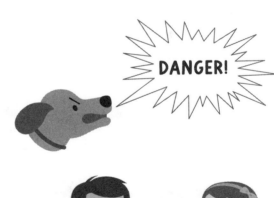

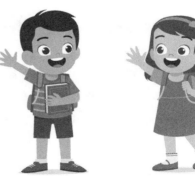

Take turns answering these questions with your adult partner. After hearing each other's responses, take a moment to compliment each other for bravely discussing this important topic.

- How can you tell if your guard dog is barking at something that's not really dangerous?

- How does having a guard dog sometimes make things harder for you?

- Can you remember a time when your guard dog thought you were in danger, but you were actually safe and sound?

By completing this activity, you have earned a

Great job!

★ Take a Brave Point from the storage bag.

★ On the back of the Brave Point, write down (or have your adult partner write down) one thing you learned by completing the activity.

★ Place the Brave Point in your supercool Brave Points Bank.

ACTIVITY 5

Bark Translator

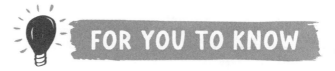

FOR YOU TO KNOW

Your guard dog's warnings, or barks, tell you what could go wrong. Your guard dog wants you to stay safe, so it might make you run, fight, hide, or do anything to survive in a situation that it believes is dangerous for you.

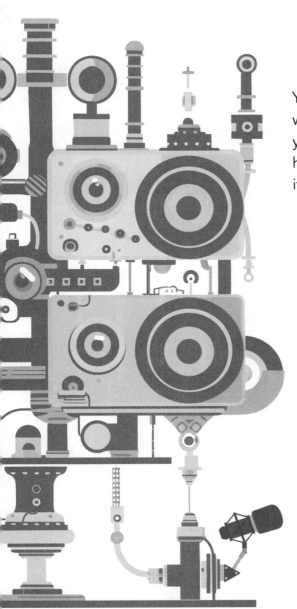

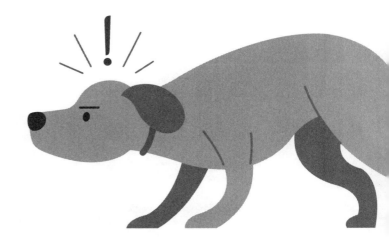

FOR YOU TO DO ☆

Think about a time when your guard dog was being too protective and telling you there was danger, but everything was actually okay. Answer the following questions:

WHERE WAS I?	
WHAT WAS I DOING?	
WHAT ELSE DO I REMEMBER ABOUT WHAT WAS GOING ON?	

Fill in the bubbles with the warnings your guard dog barked at you.

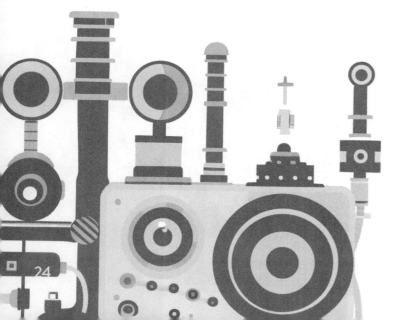

24

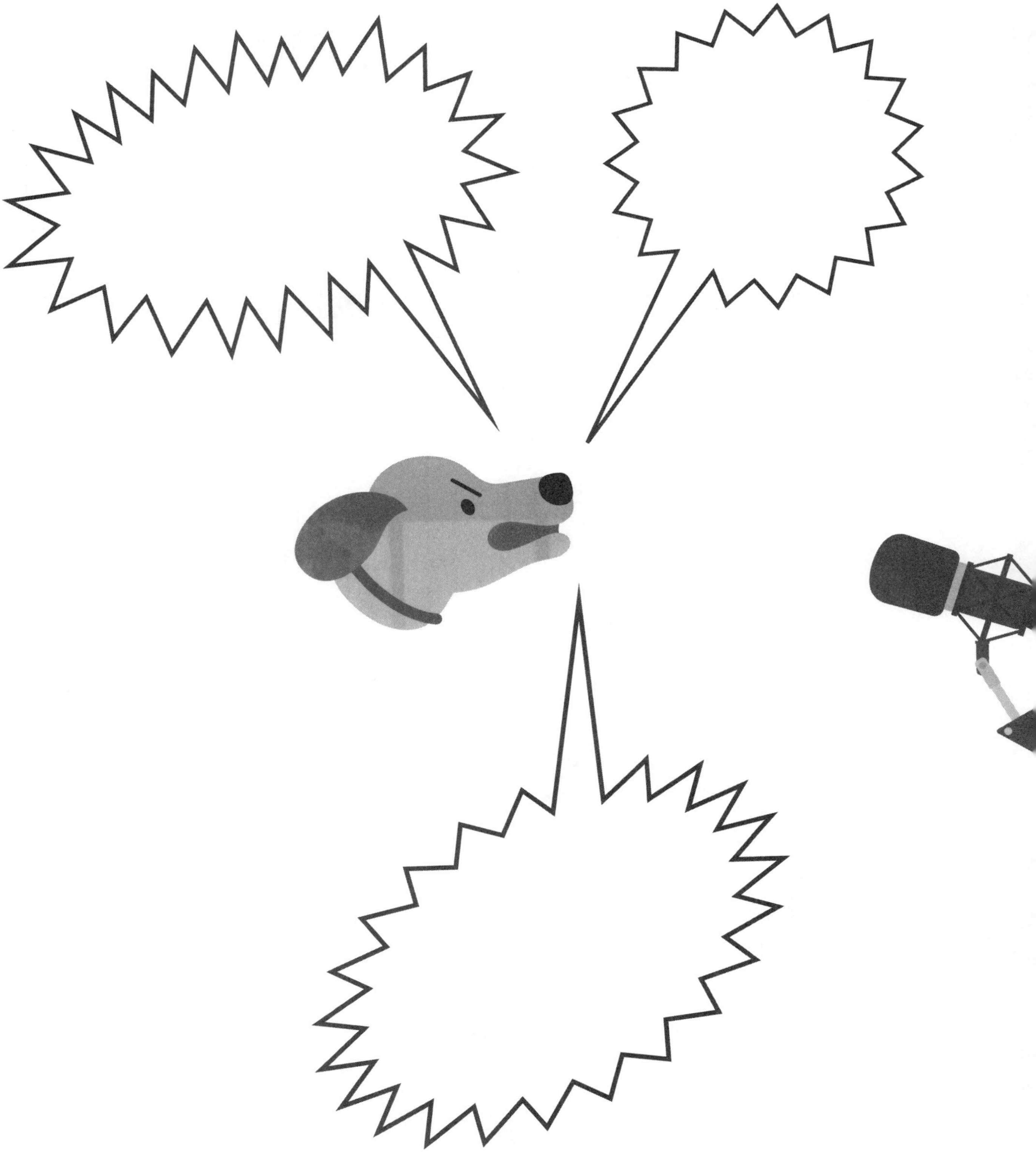

For example, Amir had to go to the doctor to get a checkup, and he started worrying about having to get a shot. Here's what he wrote down:

WHERE WAS I?	In my room...and then I ran into my parents' room once I got really scared.
WHAT WAS I DOING?	Lying in bed, trying to fall asleep.
WHAT ELSE DO I REMEMBER ABOUT WHAT WAS GOING ON?	I was thinking about how Zoe told me she got a shot the last time she went to the doctor and how painful and awful she said it was.

Here are the warnings that Amir's guard dog barked:

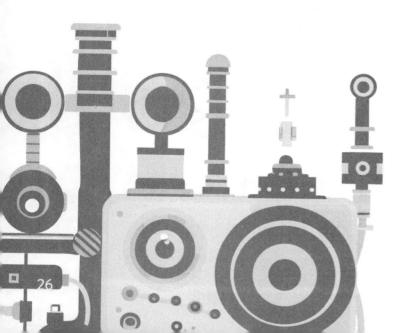

The shots are going to be painful.

It's going to be scary.

It's going to be awful.

27

Take turns answering these questions with your adult partner. After hearing each other's responses, take a moment to compliment each other for bravely discussing this important topic.

- Describe a recent situation where you felt afraid. What kinds of thoughts was your guard dog causing you to have?

- Was your guard dog right? Did the bad things it warned you about actually happen?

By completing this activity, you have earned a

Great job!

★ **Take a Brave Point from the storage bag.**

★ **On the back of the Brave Point, write down (or have your adult partner write down) one thing you learned by completing the activity.**

★ **Place the Brave Point in your supercool Brave Points Bank.**

What Breed Is Your Guard Dog?

Just like you, your guard dog is unique and has special qualities that makes it different from other people's guard dogs.

Here are some guard dogs that work really hard to keep their owners safe. But remember, there are many different types of guard dogs out there. Your guard dog might be a mix of these different types. Your guard dog has its own unique bark to warn you about any possible danger you might face.

The first guard dog you are going to meet is the Shy Guy Shih Tzu.

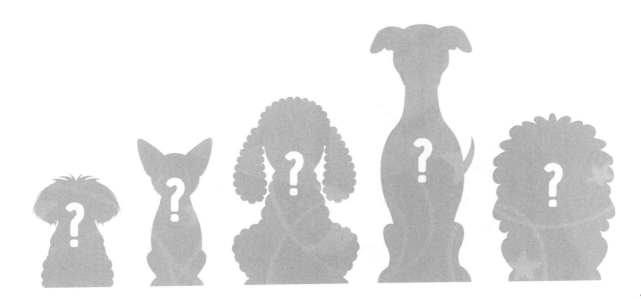

Shy Guy Shih Tzus tend to fear:

- not being liked

- doing something embarrassing

- going to parties or crowded places

- speaking in class

- speaking to a less-familiar adult, such as a waitress at a restaurant

- eating in front of others

- changing clothes in front of others

- using public bathrooms

- speaking on a telephone

- entering a classroom or activity late

- writing or drawing in front of others.

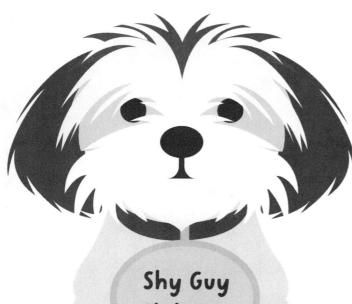

Shy Guy Shih Tzu

The next guard dog you are going to meet is the **Keep Me Close Chihuahua**.

Keep Me Close Chihuahuas tend to fear:

- being left home alone

- getting lost or separated from your family

- something bad happening to your family

- sleeping alone

- going to school or being anywhere away from your parents.

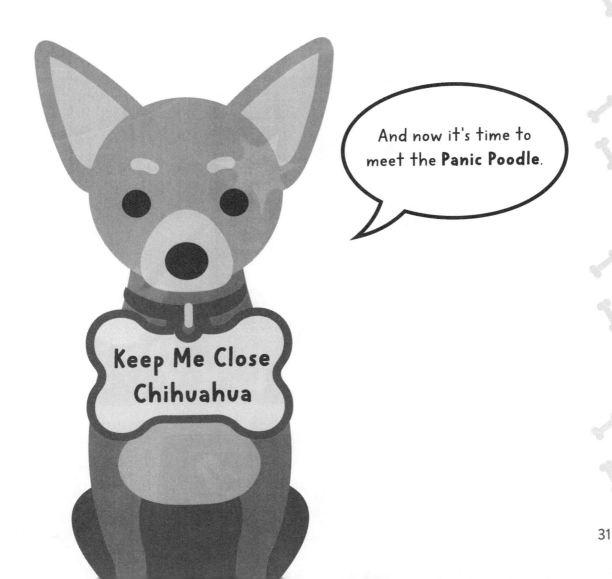

Keep Me Close Chihuahua

And now it's time to meet the **Panic Poodle**.

Panic Poodles tend to fear:

- scary feelings in your body

- your heart beating too fast

- feeling dizzy

- feeling shaky

- tummy aches and feeling unwell

- feeling like things are not real

- feeling warm or sweaty

- having a choking feeling or difficulty breathing

- having a panic attack.

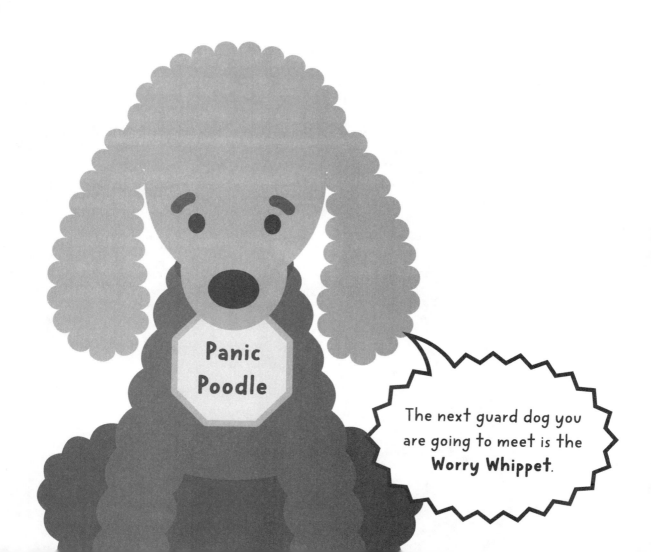

Panic Poodle

The next guard dog you are going to meet is the **Worry Whippet**.

Worry Whippets tend to worry about:

- doing well in school or sports

- needing to know the plan for the day

- the future or things that have already happened

- if family is going to be safe and healthy

- being as good as other kids

- doing something while someone else is watching.

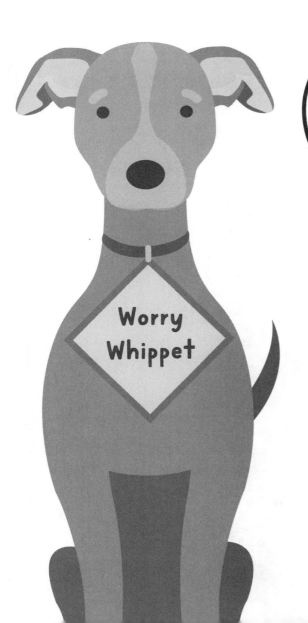

Worry Whippet

It's time for you to meet the cute, furry, and always watchful **Checking Chow Chow**.

Checking Chow Chows tend to worry about:

- not understanding things well enough

- something going terribly wrong unless you do exactly what they ask you to do

- not being sure enough that everything will be okay

- forgetting to do something important

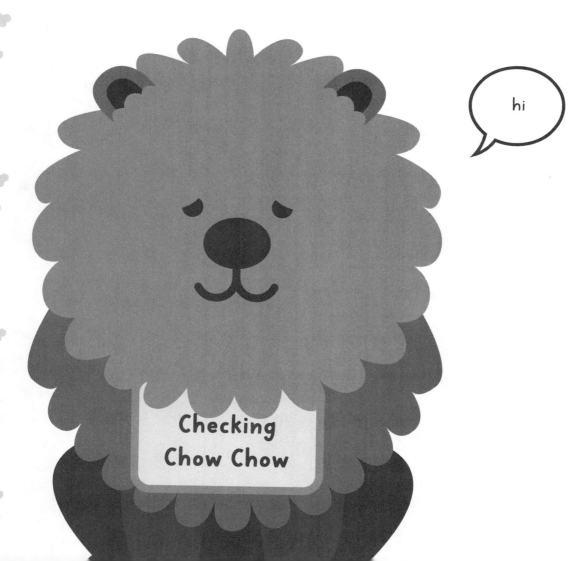

GUARD DOG PATROL

Always Ready to Protect You From Danger...
Even When There Is No Danger to Protect You From

Don't get left alone!

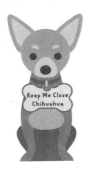

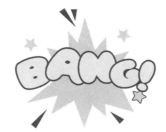

Don't do anything embarrasing!

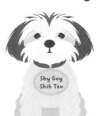

Do what I tell you to do or else something bad will happen!

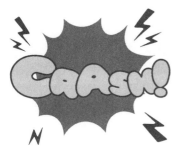

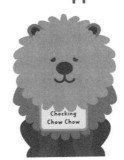

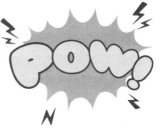

Something awful is going to happen!

Make sure you don't make a mistake!

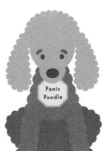

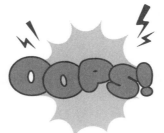

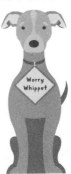

Now tell us, what are we missing?

Does your guard dog have any other worries we have not discussed?

- _____

- _____

- _____

When your guard dog is worried about these other things, what do they bark at you?

- _____

- _____

★ FOR YOU TO DO ★

Let's learn more about what makes your guard dog feel scared and worried.

From the list below, check off the warnings your guard dog barks at you.

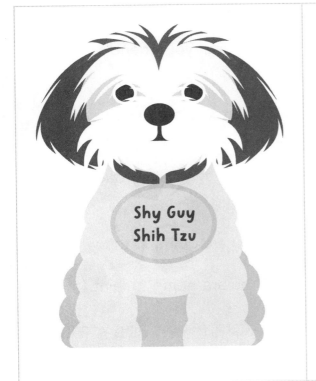

Shy Guy
Shih Tzu

◯ "People don't like you."

◯ "Everyone thinks you are weird."

◯ "You will embarrass yourself if you speak in class."

◯ "Going to that party will be awful because no one is going to want to hang out with you."

◯ "Everyone is looking at you and can tell how awkward you are."

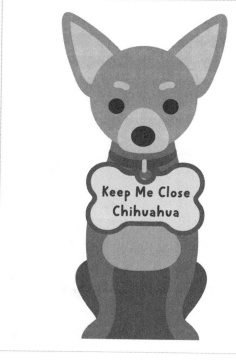

Keep Me Close
Chihuahua

○ "You are not safe unless you can see your parents."

○ "You will keep feeling scared until you are with your parents."

○ "You can't fall asleep without your parents."

○ "It will be terrible to sleepover at your friend's house."

○ "It is too scary to be alone."

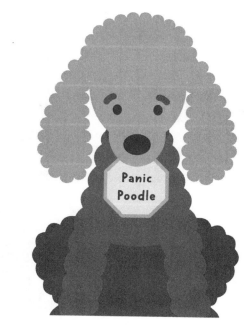

Panic
Poodle

○ "Something really bad is happening."

○ "You are going to throw up."

○ "You are going to faint."

○ "There is something wrong with you."

○ "You are in danger."

38

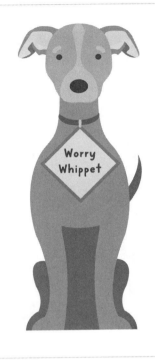

Worry
Whippet

○ "You are going to fail the test."

○ "There is going to be a terrible storm."

○ "If you make a mistake, everything will be ruined."

○ "Things are not going to work out."

○ "Something bad could happen to your parents."

Checking
Chow Chow

○ "You need to do that again or else something bad will happen."

○ "You are going to keep feeling awful until you check again that everything is okay."

○ "You need to check to make sure you understand."

○ "You need to reread or rewrite that to make sure you did not make a mistake."

○ "You need to ask your parents to say that again or else something bad will happen."

OTHER GUARD DOG WARNINGS:

○ _____

○ _____

○ _____

○ _____

○ _____

Count the total number of barks you checked off for each guard dog type to see what unique combination of breeds that you have.

GUARD DOG TYPE	# OF BARKS
Shy Guy Shih Tzu	
Keep Me Close Chihuahua	
Panic Poodle	
Worry Whippet	
Checking Chow Chow	
Other	

Draw a picture of your guard dog. Be sure to include all of its unique qualities.

Take turns discussing your answers to the following questions with your adult partner. After hearing each other's responses, take a moment to compliment each other for bravely discussing this important topic.

- What is your unique combination of breeds?

- Is your guard dog more of one breed than another?

- What is the name of your guard dog?

- Can you draw a picture of your guard dog?

By completing this activity, you have earned a

Great job!

★ **Take a Brave Point from the storage bag.**

★ **On the back of the Brave Point, write down (or have your adult partner write down) one thing you learned by completing the activity.**

★ **Place the Brave Point in your supercool Brave Points Bank.**

ACTIVITY
7

How to Train Your Guard Dog

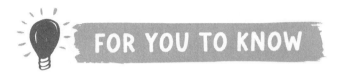

FOR YOU TO KNOW

As you now know, just because your guard dog is barking does not mean anything is actually wrong or bad. But all that extra barking sure can be distracting and make it hard to hear other important things. The good news is that your guard dog is not only loyal and oh-so eager to protect you, it is also highly trainable. You can train your guard dog to pay attention to you. Your guard dog can learn to calm down when you send a signal that it was just a false alarm and you are actually safe and sound.

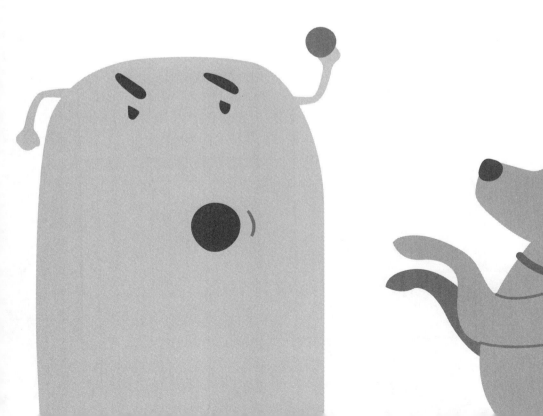

FOR YOU TO DO ⭐

This exercise will teach you how to train your guard dog to listen to you, to bark less, and to stay calm.

STEP 1: ATTENTION

Think of a word you can use to get your guard dog's attention. What word can you say to get your guard dog to focus on you instead of on the false alarm? Some of our friends picked words such as:

- Sit

- Here

- Look

What word or words can you use to get your guard dog's attention?

STEP 2: CALM DOWN

Calmly tell your guard dog, "You can stop barking, you are safe and sound, and there is nothing wrong."

What other ways can you tell your guard dog the coast is clear and it's safe to stop barking?

STEP 3: PRAISE

When your guard dog calms down and stops barking, praise it for listening and being a good dog!

Some of our friends have said things like the phrases below when their guard dog listens to them and stops barking:

- Good dog!

- Great job!

- I am proud of you!

What will you say to praise your guard dog for being such a good dog and listening to you and stopping barking?

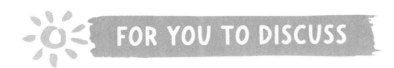

FOR YOU TO DISCUSS

Take turns discussing your answers to the following questions with your adult partner. After hearing each other's responses, take a moment to compliment each other for bravely discussing this important topic.

- Do you find it easy or hard to get your guard dog to pay attention to you?

- What helps you to get your guard dog's attention, and what makes it harder?

- Do you ever get frustrated with your guard dog's barking? If so, does anger make your guard dog stop barking or bark even louder?

- Do you think your guard dog deserves praise when it listens to you and stops barking?

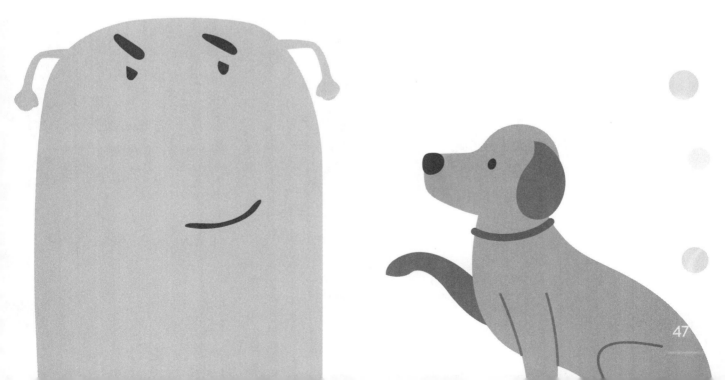

By completing this activity, you have earned a

Great job!

★ Take a Brave Point from the storage bag.

★ On the back of the Brave Point, write down (or have your adult partner write down) one thing you learned by completing the activity.

★ Place the Brave Point in your supercool Brave Points Bank.

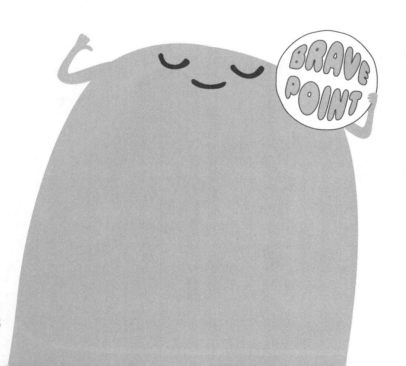

ACTIVITY 8

Scary Feeling IScream Shop

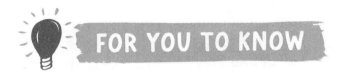

When you feel scared, different feelings can pop up inside you! It's important to pay attention to these feelings as soon as they appear. The sooner you catch your guard dog getting worked up, the easier it is to calm it down. If your guard dog is already in full panic mode, it will have a hard time listening to you or doing anything else except barking loudly to warn you of danger. In that state, it's really hard to have fun, relax, or pretty much enjoy anything at all.

To catch your guard dog from getting into panic mode early, you need to become aware of the different flavors of fear. By doing this, you'll get better at noticing the early signs of fear. For example, you might notice a nauseous feeling when you're scared. Then, you can ask yourself, "Is there really something bad happening, or is this just my guard dog having a false alarm?" This helps you decide whether to react or not, and it gives you more control over your feelings and actions.

Welcome to the IScream Scary Feeling Ice Cream Shop, the yummiest scary feeling ice cream shop in the world. If you could scoop up all the different "scary feeling" flavors you have when you're afraid, which flavors would you choose?

1. Circle the "Scary Feeling Flavors" that describe how you feel when your guard dog is barking at you.

ISCREAM
SCARY FEELING ICE CREAM SHOP

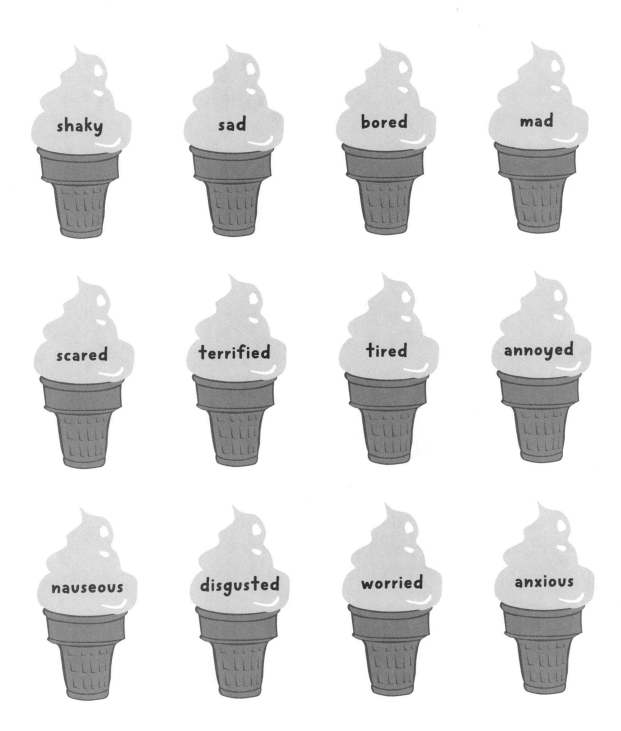

2. Write down or have your adult partner write down other scary feeling flavors that are not included on the main menu. Special requests are encouraged at the IScream Scary Feeling Ice Cream Shop!

CREATE YOUR OWN
ISCREAM FLAVORS

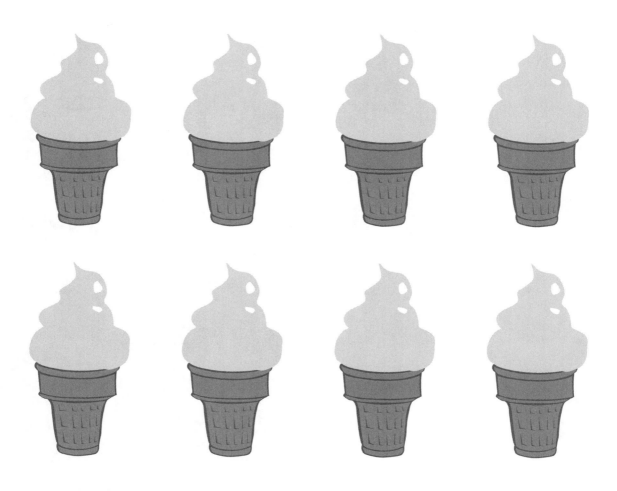

3. Think about a time when you felt really scared. What was happening? Now imagine how your body felt in that moment. Think about all the uncomfortable, yucky, and crummy feelings you were experiencing. Write them down.

4. Draw a picture of your scary feeling iscream cone for that tough moment. Add a scoop for each scary feeling you had. Write the feeling in or next to the scoop. You can make this iscream cone as big as you want, so pile on scoops of those scary feeling flavors! There are no limits to the number of scary feelings any of us have when we're afraid.

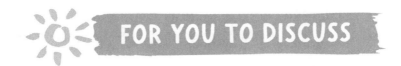

FOR YOU TO DISCUSS

Take turns discussing your answers to the following questions with your adult partner. After hearing each other's responses, take a moment to compliment each other for bravely discussing this important topic.

- Tell me about a recent time you were afraid.

- What fear flavors were on your iscream cone?

Discuss with your adult partner:

- Which scary feeling flavors do you have that your adult partner does not have?

- Which scary feeling flavors does your adult partner have that you don't have?

By completing this activity, you have earned a

Great job!

★ Take a Brave Point from the storage bag.

★ On the back of the Brave Point, write down (or have your adult partner write down) one thing you learned by completing the activity.

★ Place the Brave Point in your supercool Brave Points Bank.

ACTIVITY
9

Your Body on Fear

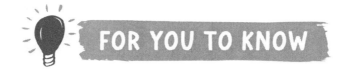

FOR YOU TO KNOW

When your guard dog senses possible danger, your body goes into what is called the 3F mode, the fight-flight-freeze mode. It's like a superpower that your body switches on to help you deal with danger.

When your guard dog thinks you are in danger when you are actually safe and sound, it can feel yucky to have all that extra power flowing through your body. It's like standing at the starting line of a race, ready to zip forward, but no one is starting the race. You are just standing there all revved up with nowhere to go.

These uncomfortable feelings are your body's way of making you stronger and faster, like a supercharged version of yourself ready to do what it takes to escape from or fight off danger.

You definitely don't want to get rid of these helpful superpowers because they are there to keep you safe. But you do need to learn to notice when your guard dog has set off your body's 3F response so you can see if the response is needed or not.

Have you ever been scared and noticed your heart beating fast? Maybe your stomach felt funny, and then you thought, *Oh no, I feel terrible, there must be something wrong with me!* That thought can make you even more scared, and then, guess what? Your heart races even faster and your stomach feels even ickier! It's like being stuck in a loop of fear. But here's the cool part—understanding these feelings of fear is like cracking a special code. Once you crack the fear code, you can break free from the fear loop and start feeling better.

FEAR OF FEAR FERRIS WHEEL

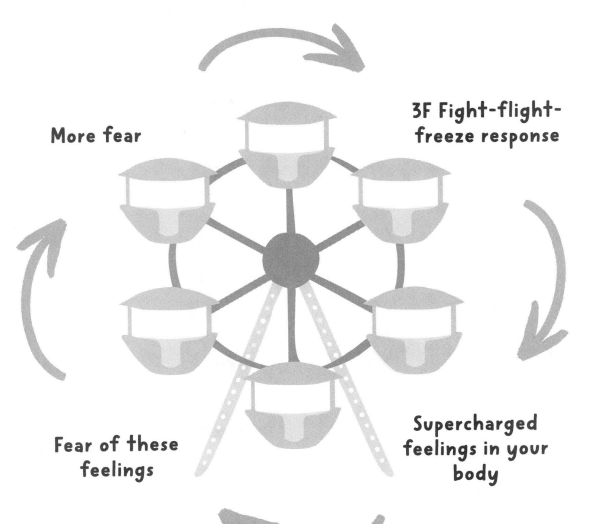

More fear

3F Fight-flight-freeze response

Fear of these feelings

Supercharged feelings in your body

YOUR SUPERCHARGED BODY IN FIGHT-FLIGHT-FREEZE MODE	HOW THIS HELPS PROTECT YOU FROM DANGER
Faster heart rate	When you feel scared, your heart beats faster and harder. Your heart pumps more blood to your muscles, giving you extra strength and energy to fight or run away from danger.
Faster breathing	When your guard dog senses danger, your breathing gets faster. Your body does this to bring in more oxygen, which is like fuel for your muscles and brain. It helps you be more alert and ready to take action if you need to.
Sweaty	Fear can make your body feel sweaty. Sweating cools your body off so you don't overheat. Plus, it is helpful to be slippery if an angry predator is trying to grab hold of you.

Upset stomach	Sometimes, fear can give you a funny feeling in your stomach, like butterflies fluttering around. This sensation is caused by your body redirecting blood away from your stomach to other parts of your body that are more important in helping you run, fight, or hide, such as muscles in your arms and legs. After all, this is no time to digest a big meal when you are about to be someone else's meal!
Shaking	When you're scared, you might notice your hands or legs get a bit shaky. This happens because your body is getting ready to react quickly. Extra blood is being sent to your arms and legs so you can be supercharged and ready to run, fight, or hide your way past danger.

Difficult time thinking clearly	When your body is in fight-flight-freeze mode, it redirects blood flow from your brain to your muscles associated with being able to run and fight, such as your arms and legs. Your guard dog does not want you to waste time thinking when you could be taking action to escape (make-believe) danger.

1. Where do you feel fear in your body? Color in the areas in the figure below where fear sensations most often show up for you.

MY BODY ON FEAR

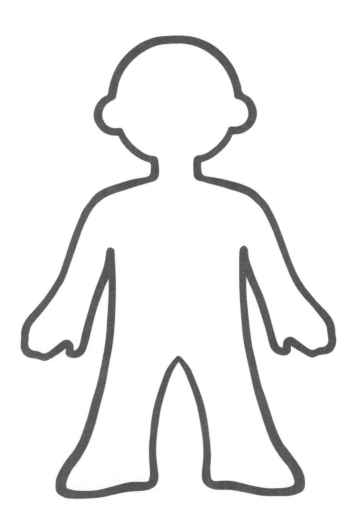

2. Think of a recent time you felt afraid and circle the sensations of fear that you experienced:

- Faster heart rate

- Faster breathing

- Increase in sweating

- Upset stomach

- Shaking

- Difficult time thinking clearly

- Other: _____

3. For each of these sensations of fear, write down why your body feels this way. Use your own words to explain what is causing the uncomfortable feelings and how they are actually part of your 3F response to make you a supercharged version of yourself, to protect you from danger.

The next time you are feeling some or all of the sensations associated with fear in your body, review these notes and remind yourself why you are feeling what you are feeling.

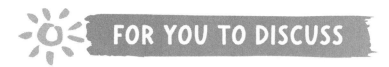

FOR YOU TO DISCUSS

Take turns discussing your answers to the following questions with your adult partner. After hearing each other's responses, take a moment to compliment each other for bravely discussing this important topic.

- Have you ever been afraid of what your body feels like when your guard dog is barking at you?

- Were you surprised to learn that your body feels that way because it is preparing you to survive DANGER?

By completing this activity, you have earned a

Great job!

★ Take a Brave Point from the storage bag.

★ On the back of the Brave Point, write down (or have your adult partner write down) one thing you learned by completing the activity.

★ Place the Brave Point in your supercool Brave Points Bank.

ACTIVITY 10

Breathing Pop It

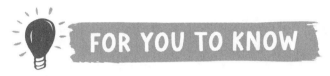

FOR YOU TO KNOW

A really helpful way to calm down your guard dog is slow breathing. Slow breathing signals your body to calm down your brain. And it is as simple as it sounds. All you need to do is two minutes of slow breathing and your body will shift from fear mode to relaxation mode.

By taking a series of slow, gentle breaths, you are sending a signal from your body to your guard dog that the coast is clear and it is safe to return to a state of calm and peace.

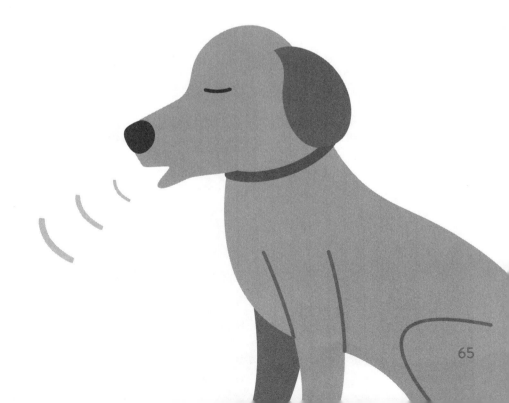

65

Tap the POP IT on the following page while following the instructions to breathe in, hold, and breathe out.

The object of the game is to tap all the numbers without skipping or missing any.

Note: Nine rounds of Tap It Square Breathing should take around two minutes to complete.

TAP IT SQUARE BREATHING

Breathe in
Hold
Breathe Out

ROUND 1

ROUND 2

ROUND 3

Breathe in
Hold
Breathe Out

ROUND 4

ROUND 5

ROUND 6

Breathe in
Hold
Breathe Out

ROUND 7

ROUND 8

ROUND 9

67

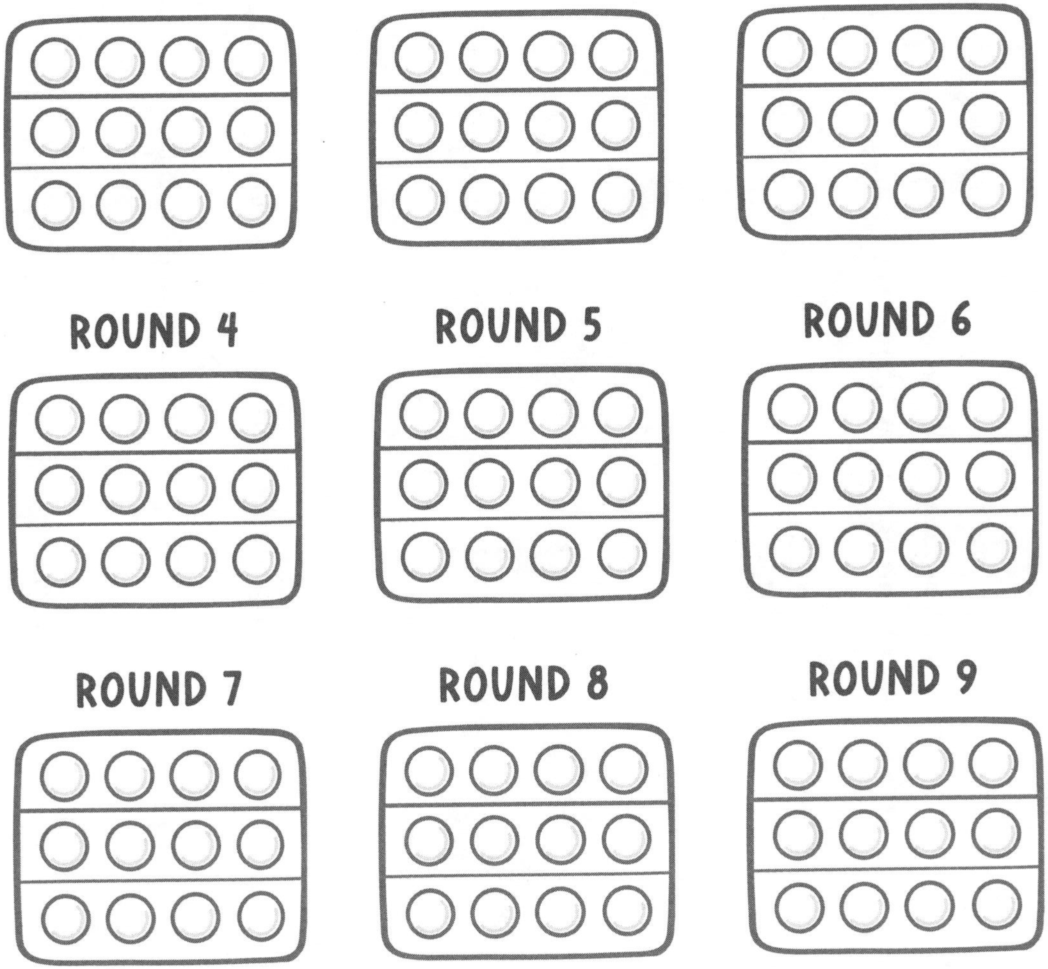

Take turns discussing your answers to the following questions with your adult partner. After hearing each other's responses, take a moment to compliment each other for bravely discussing this important topic.

● How many rounds of Tap It Square Breathing were you able to complete?

● Did any of the rounds feel different as you kept going?

● How did you feel after playing the Tap It Square Breathing game?

By completing this activity, you have earned a

Great job!

★ **Take a Brave Point from the storage bag.**

★ **On the back of the Brave Point, write down (or have your adult partner write down) one thing you learned by completing the activity.**

★ **Place the Brave Point in your supercool Brave Points Bank.**

Thought-Feeling-Action Loopty-Loop

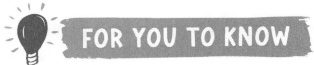

FOR YOU TO KNOW

What you think changes how you feel, which changes what you do. Round and round you go on the Thought-Feeling-Action Loopty-Loop.

For example, if your mom reminds you that you have a checkup with your doctor after school, there are different options for which Thought-Feeling-Action Loopty-Loop you ride.

OPTION 1:

1. Thought: *This is going to be awful.*

2. Feeling: Scared.

3. Action: You yell at Mom and tell her she is so mean for ruining your day and making you go to this appointment.

OPTION 2:

1. Thought: *I may not like going to the doctor, but it always ends up fine.*

2. Feeling: Slightly cranky but calm.

3. Action: You tell your mom you are not looking forward to the appointment but know it is important to go.

Changing your thoughts can change how you feel for the better. If your big feeling gets smaller, you will probably feel braver to do things that are helpful for you and others.

69

FOR YOU TO DO ☆

1. Imagine you are going to a sleepover at a friend's house for the first time. Write down the thoughts, feelings, and actions you could have if you wanted to go on the scariest Thought-Action-Feeling Loopty-Loop.

A scary thought you might have: _____

_____

A scary feeling you might have: _____

_____

A scary action you could take: _____

_____

Fill in the blanks on the calm loopty-loop.

SCARY THOUGHT

SCARY ACTION

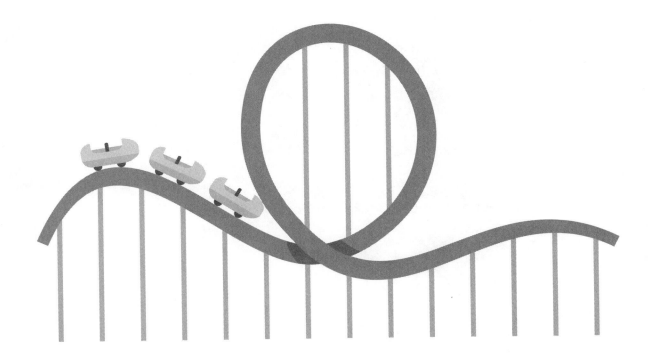

SCARY FEELING

Phew, what a ride! However, you can make the loops less scary and frightening and stop them from going too high and too fast.

2. What kind of thoughts, feelings, and actions could make the loopty-loop less bumpy and rough?

A calming thought you might have: _____

_____

A calming feeling you might have: _____

_____

A calming action you could take: _____

_____

Fill in the blanks on the calm loopty-loop.

CALMING THOUGHT

CALMING ACTION

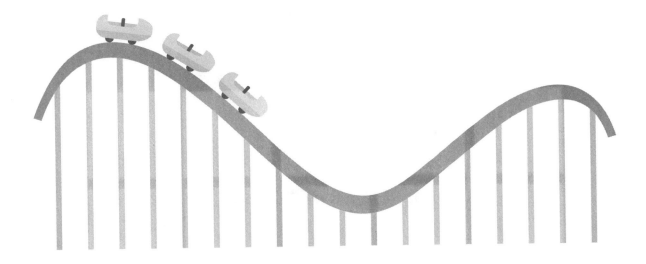

CALMING FEELING

☀ FOR YOU TO DISCUSS

Take turns discussing your answers to the following questions with your adult partner. After hearing each other's responses, take a moment to compliment each other for bravely discussing this important topic.

- Can you think of a time when you started feeling sad but then something made you feel happy? What turned your feelings around?

- Think about a time you did something when you were feeling upset to make yourself feel better. What brave action did you take to make things better?

- Tell me about a time a tricky thought tried to make you feel scared. How did you change your thoughts to feel calmer and more relaxed?

By completing this activity, you have earned a

Great job!

★ **Take a Brave Point from the storage bag.**

★ **On the back of the Brave Point, write down (or have your adult partner write down) one thing you learned by completing the activity.**

★ **Place the Brave Point in your supercool Brave Points Bank.**

Your Dream Pizza

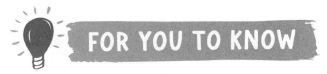

FOR YOU TO KNOW

You can imagine your life as a delicious pizza with different slices representing important parts of your life. If you felt less scared and more confident to do all the things you want to do, what fun toppings would you put on your pizza?

FOR YOU TO DO

Imagine all the fun things you would like to do if your guard dog were quieter and you felt less afraid. Use your imagination to dream big and think about the different exciting experiences you would like to be having. This is a time to imagine endless possibilities and have fun, without worrying about how you will make them happen. Let your imagination run wild with all the amazing things you could do!

Fill in each slice of this dream pizza with wishes for what you would like your life to look like if fear and worries were no longer getting in your way.

zzzz...

THE FUN I COULD HAVE

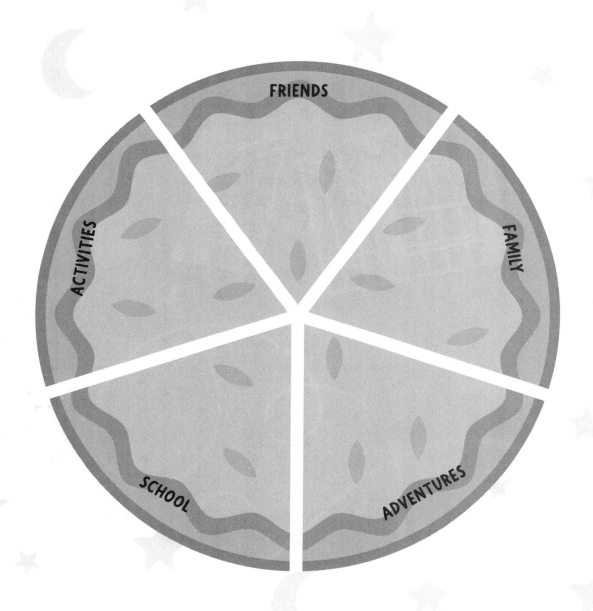

THE FUN I COULD HAVE

For example, Olivia's dream pizza looks this:

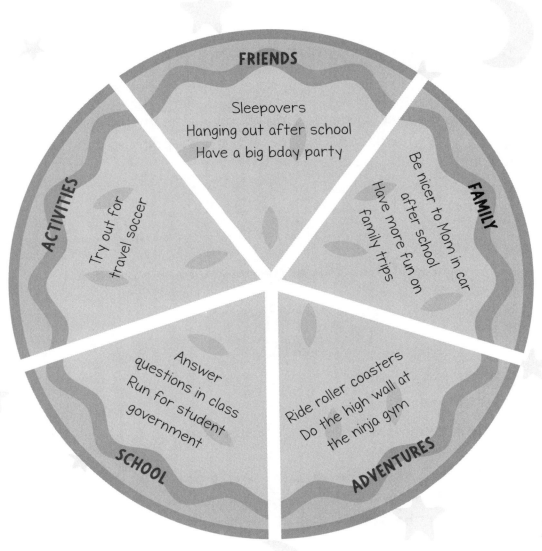

FRIENDS

Sleepovers
Hanging out after school
Have a big bday party

FAMILY

Be nicer to Mom in car after school
Have more fun on family trips

ACTIVITIES

Try out for travel soccer

SCHOOL

Answer questions in class
Run for student government

ADVENTURES

Ride roller coasters
Do the high wall at the ninja gym

Take turns discussing your answers to the following questions with your adult partner. After hearing each other's responses, take a moment to compliment each other for bravely discussing this important topic.

- How does your guard dog block you from adding fun toppings to your dream pizza?

- If you could only add one fun topping to your dream pizza, which one would you add first? What makes this fun topping so important to you?

By completing this activity, you have earned a

Great job!

★ Take a Brave Point from the storage bag.

★ On the back of the Brave Point, write down (or have your adult partner write down) one thing you learned by completing the activity.

★ Place the Brave Point in your supercool Brave Points Bank.

ACTIVITY

13

Focus Pocus

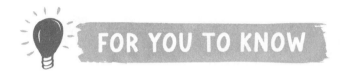

FOR YOU TO KNOW

Fears and worries don't have to completely go away for you to have freedom from them. By taking a step back and looking at things in a different way, you'll find that your guard dog's barks become softer, and your worries and fears won't take as much of your energy. This gives you the power to focus on fun things happening around you instead of feeling stuck and locked into your worry thoughts.

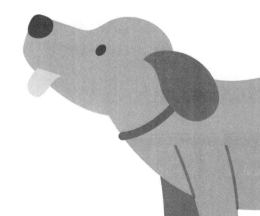

FOR YOU TO DO

1. Gather supplies: 1 pencil or pen, sticky notes.

2. Think of a recent situation when your guard dog was having a false-alarm moment and warning you of danger when all was actually okay.

3. On one side of a sticky note, write down one of the warnings your guard dog was barking at you.

4. On the other side of the sticky note, draw a picture of the danger your guard dog was warning you about.

5. Place the sticky note over one of your eyes and notice how much else you can see when you are allowing your guard dog to boss you around. How much of your view is taken over by this fear?

6. Next, remove the sticky note from your face and place it on a wall across the room.

7. Now look at the worry thought and see how small it looks. Can you look at the worry thought and still see other things happening around you?

Take turns answering these questions with your adult partner. After hearing each other's responses, take a moment to compliment each other for bravely discussing this important topic.

- When have you had a worry thought stuck in your brain, making it hard for you to pay attention to anything else?

- When you are having this worry thought, does it make it difficult for you to pay attention to other parts of your life?

- What helps you get unstuck from your worry thoughts so you can pay more attention to other parts of your life?

By completing this activity, you have earned a

Great job!

★ **Take a Brave Point from the storage bag.**

★ **On the back of the Brave Point, write down (or have your adult partner write down) one thing you learned by completing the activity.**

★ **Place the Brave Point in your supercool Brave Points Bank.**

Hoo Hoo? Your Wise Owl, That's Who!

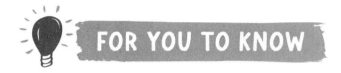

FOR YOU TO KNOW

Just like your Feeling Brain can be compared to a guard dog, always ready to protect you, your Thinking Brain can be compared to a wise owl. Your wise owl is there to guide you and help you solve problems.

Your wise owl is like a helpful friend. This friend reminds you to think carefully and collect all the facts before taking action. They make sure you have all the important information. Your wise owl is there to help you make smart choices and do things in a way that will be best for you.

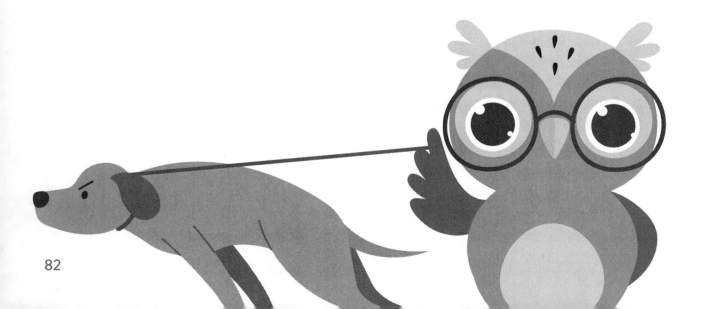

WISE OWL JOB DESCRIPTION

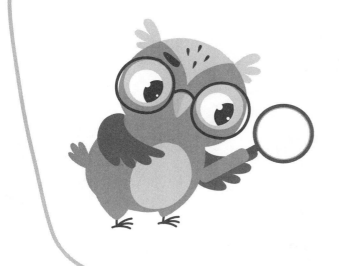

1. Search for clues.

2. Understand the facts.

3. Take a bit of time to think and consider what to do next.

4. Share advice in a calm, unemotional way.

Your wise owl is really good at making smart decisions because it takes the time to think carefully about all the different facts and information. How does your wise owl do this? By paying close attention to everything going on around you! By watching and carefully gathering important information, you will understand more of what is going on around you.

Learning to find the right balance between your guard dog's warnings and your wise owl's advice is the best recipe to make your dream pizza a reality. By listening to both your guard dog and your wise owl, you can stay safe and live your most fun and best life.

Ellie was invited to a party that she was both excited and scared to attend. Let's take a look at what her guard dog was barking at her.

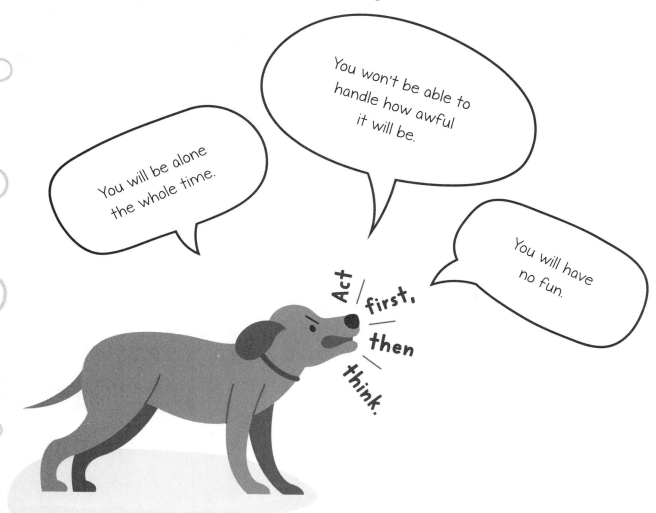

Thankfully, her wise owl was there to remind her that sometimes parties can be fun.

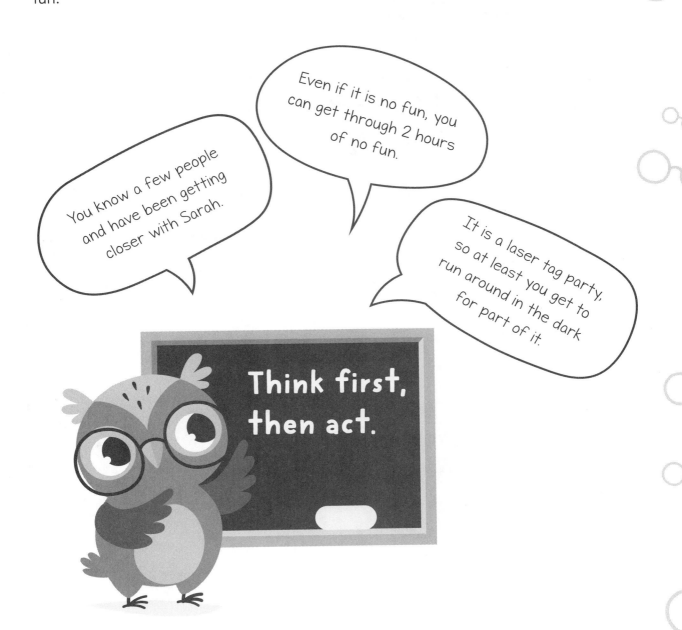

You know a few people and have been getting closer with Sarah.

Even if it is no fun, you can get through 2 hours of no fun.

It is a laser tag party, so at least you get to run around in the dark for part of it.

Think first, then act.

Ellie thought about what both her guard dog and her wise owl had to say. Then she decided to take her wise owl's advice because she didn't want to let her fears hold her back from enjoying herself. Ellie ended up going to the party and having a pretty good time (not perfect but certainly not awful).

By balancing the advice of her guard dog and wise owl, Ellie was able to enjoy a delicious, sizzling slice of her dream pizza, complete with her favorite toppings of friends and parties.

Now it's your turn!

1. Think of a recent situation when your guard dog was barking at you to warn you of danger.

2. Draw a picture of the situation your guard dog feared.

3. Write the warnings your guard dog was barking at you and what they wanted you to do.

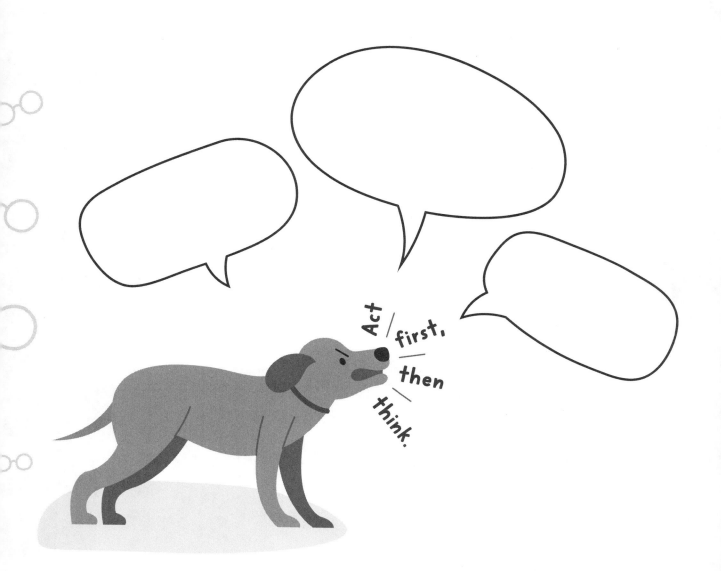

4. What advice does your wise owl have for you about how you can handle this situation?

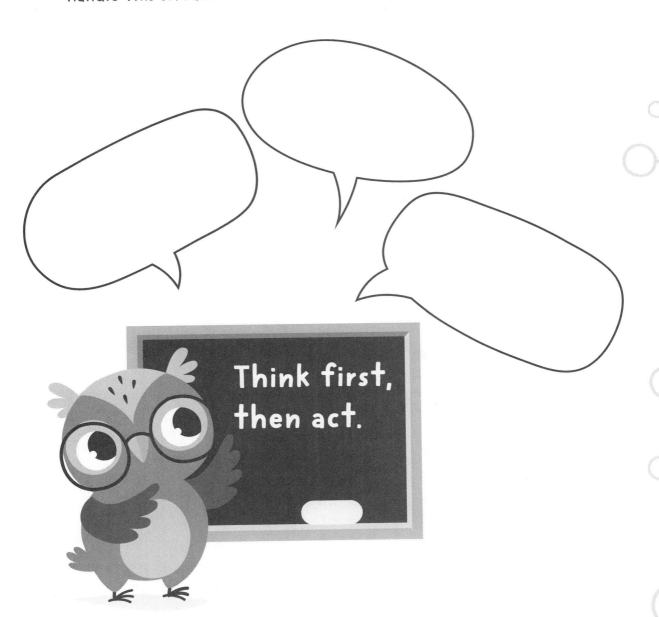

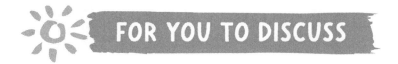

FOR YOU TO DISCUSS

Take turns answering these questions with your adult partner. After hearing each other's responses, take a moment to compliment each other for bravely discussing this important topic.

- When was your guard dog barking at you?

- What three things did your guard dog say?

1. _____

2. _____

3. _____

- What are three pieces of advice your wise owl would give you about this same situation?

1. _____

2. _____

3. _____

- Do you normally believe all the warnings your guard dog barks at you? Or do you also try to listen to your wise owl?

- Do you have any advice on how I can hear my wise owl when my guard dog is barking loudly?

By completing this activity, you have earned a

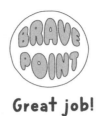

Great job!

★ Take a Brave Point from the storage bag.

★ On the back of the Brave Point, write down (or have your adult partner write down) one thing you learned by completing the activity.

★ Place the Brave Point in your supercool Brave Points Bank.

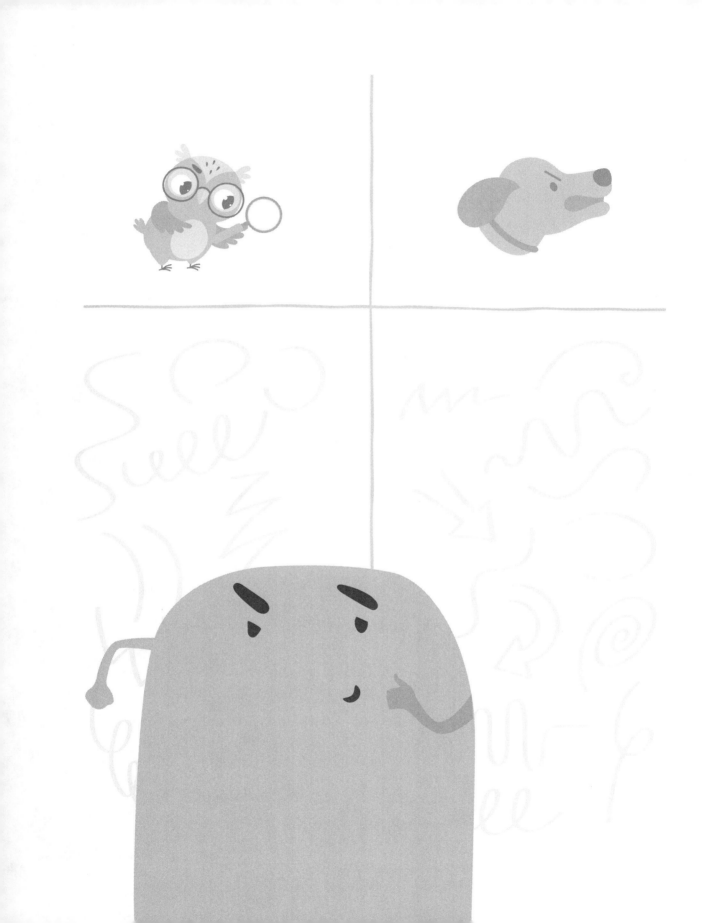

Healthy Competition

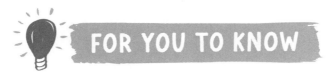

FOR YOU TO KNOW

You can think of your wise owl and your guard dog as your two very own helpful life coaches! Your guard dog is a super careful coach, always points out things that might be tricky, and suggests safe choices, saying stuff like, "Watch out!" and "Be careful!"

Your wise owl is a cool and experienced coach. It helps you figure out how to solve problems. It gives you different tips on how to reach your goals. When you're playing the game of life, your wise owl cheers you on with chants like, "You've got this," and "Keep trying!"

To be a life champion, you've got to know when to take your guard dog's cautious, careful advice and when to embrace the encouraging advice of your wise owl. That way, you'll have the best of both worlds: knowing when to play it safe and when to push yourself forward into new and exciting life adventures!

FOR YOU TO DO

For the next week, turn every stressful, challenging moment into a game with your wise owl and guard dog coaches!

Here's how:

1. **Listen up.** When faced with a tricky situation, tune in to the messages from both your wise owl and your guard dog.

2. **Decide.** Take a moment to decide whose advice you're going to follow. Are you team wise owl, ready to problem solve your way through the challenge? Or are you team guard dog, playing it safe to prevent anything bad from happening?

3. **Track your choices.** Use the following chart to mark which coach you decided to listen to each time.

4. **Count the points.** At the end of the week, tally up the points for each side. See which coach's advice and guidance you chose more often.

This fun challenge will help you discover whether you're a wise owl problem-solver or a guard dog safety enthusiast. Let the game begin and may the best coach win!

**KEEP IT GOING!
YOU GOT THIS!**

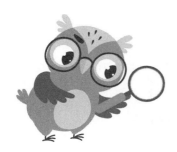

**WATCH OUT!
YOU MIGHT GET HURT!**

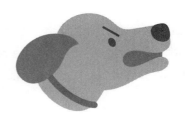

Take turns answering these questions with your adult partner. After hearing each other's responses, take a moment to compliment each other for bravely discussing this important topic.

- When did you listen to your guard dog's advice? What was going on, and what did it tell you to do?

- When did you decide to follow your wise owl's advice? What was going on, and what did it tell you to do?

- Which one do you listen to more often in tough situations: your guard dog or your wise owl? Why do you think that happens?

- Would it be helpful to get better at noticing what advice your guard dog and wise owl are offering you? Would it be helpful to choose whose advice to follow depending on what's happening? Why or why not?

By completing this activity, you have earned a

Great job!

★ Take a Brave Point from the storage bag.

★ On the back of the Brave Point, write down (or have your adult partner write down) one thing you learned by completing the activity.

★ Place the Brave Point in your supercool Brave Points Bank.

Mindfulness Express Train

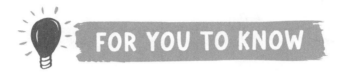

FOR YOU TO KNOW

When your guard dog barks a distracting warning message, it can take you away from a fun moment and transport you to a scary place that exists only in your imagination. The good news is that all you need to do to bring yourself back to the fun moment is to hop on the Mindfulness Express!

To ride the Mindfulness Express Train, you will focus on your five senses, journeying away from your guard dog's FALSE ALARM and back to NOW.

No tickets or planning is needed to board the Mindfulness Express. You can guide yourself away from your fears and worries and back to the fun of your current moment any time!

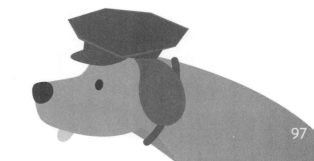

FOR YOU TO DO ★

1. Think of a recent moment when your guard dog was barking DANGER at you.

2. Spend one minute getting yourself as scared and uncomfortable as possible.

3. Draw a picture of the "scary place" your guard dog took you to.

4. Draw a picture of the "fun place" you would like the Mindfulness Express Train to take you to.

5. Ride the Mindfulness Express to bring yourself back to the current moment ("the fun place") by doing the following:

   Look around the space you are in and notice and then write down:

   - 1 thing you see

   - 1 thing you hear

   - 1 thing you can touch

   - 1 thing you smell

   - 1 thing you taste

STEP 1:
Draw a picture of the SCARY PLACE your guard dog took you to.

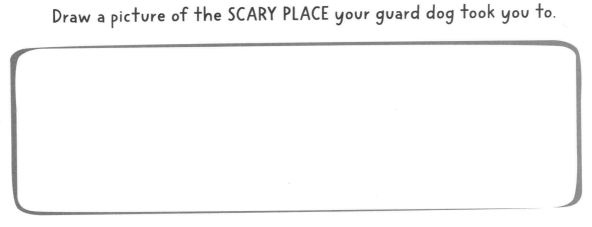

STEP 2:
Draw a picture of the FUN PLACE you would like to return back to.

STEP 3:
Ride the Mindfulness Express Train
back to the present moment.

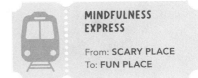

MINDFULNESS EXPRESS

From: **SCARY PLACE**
To: **FUN PLACE**

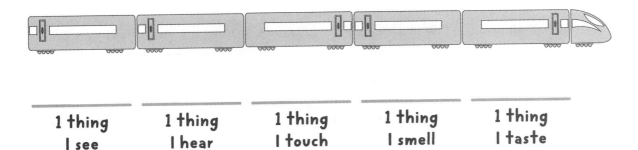

1 thing I see	1 thing I hear	1 thing I touch	1 thing I smell	1 thing I taste

Take turns answering these questions with your adult partner. After hearing each other's responses, take a moment to compliment each other for bravely discussing this important topic.

- What was it like to ride the Mindfulness Express Train?

- Was it hard to bring yourself back to the "fun place"? How hard is it for you to use your five senses to ride the Mindfulness Express Train, on a scale of 0 to 10, with 0 being a piece of cake and 10 being extremely difficult?

- How many times did you need to use the five senses? Did you notice times when you were back at the "scary place" without noticing?

By completing this activity, you have earned a

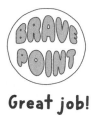

Great job!

★ Take a Brave Point from the storage bag.

★ On the back of the Brave Point, write down (or have your adult partner write down) one thing you learned by completing the activity.

★ Place the Brave Point in your supercool Brave Points Bank.

Mindful Coloring

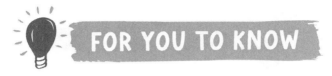

FOR YOU TO KNOW

No matter how well you train your guard dog, sometimes it barks loudly, thinking there's trouble when everything is actually okay. But guess what? You can get really good at ignoring those loud barks and focusing on something fun. If you ever get caught up in the loud, distracting false-alarm sound, all you have to do is hop back on the Mindfulness Express Train and quickly transport yourself back to the Here and Now. By practicing bringing your attention back to the present moment instead of getting stuck in worry thoughts, you'll feel less stressed and have more fun!

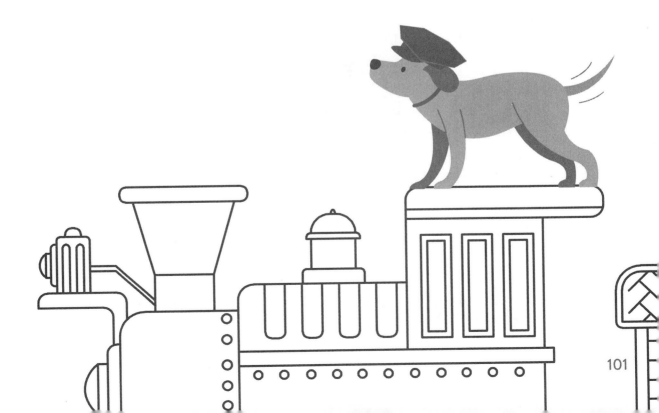

1. Gather supplies: Pencil or pen, sticky note or small piece of paper, markers or crayons.

2. Think about a guard dog moment: Remember a time when your guard dog barked danger messages at you, warning you of all the things that could go wrong.

3. Write down the warning message your guard dog gave you.

4. Draw a picture of the "danger" on the other side of the paper.

5. Now it is time to ride the mindfulness express train and practice placing your attention on the current moment. Together with your adult partner, color in the following picture.

- Pay attention to the bright colors, the sound of your markers, what it feels like to hold the marker in your hand, and all the fun details of this coloring experience.

- When your mind wanders off and starts thinking about the danger message your guard dog barked at you or anything else, gently bring it back to this fun moment of coloring in this page with your adult partner.

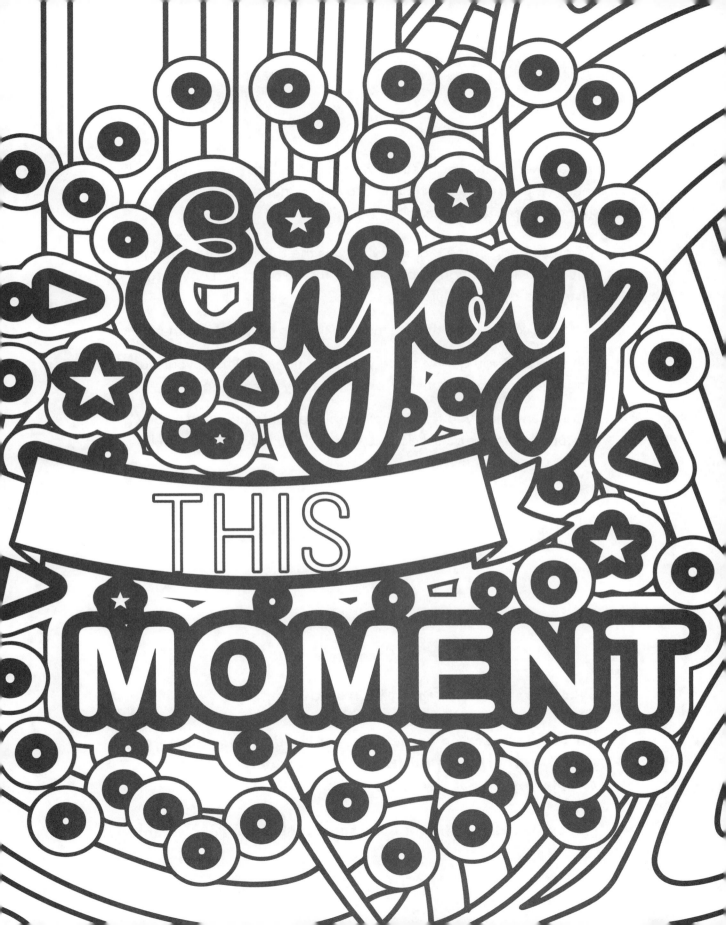

☀ FOR YOU TO DISCUSS

Take turns answering these questions with your adult partner. After hearing each other's responses, take a moment to compliment each other for bravely discussing this important topic.

- When coloring in the picture, what was the trickiest part of trying to put as much attention as possible on the coloring and not getting distracted by your guard dog's barks?

- Are there certain barks that are more distracting for you than other barks?

- What helped you gently guide your attention away from your guard dog's barks and place it back on our activity of coloring?

- Is there anything you try to remind yourself of to help you to get unstuck from your guard dog's barks and bring your attention back to our coloring activity?

By completing this activity, you have earned a

Great job!

★ Take a Brave Point from the storage bag.

★ On the back of the Brave Point, write down (or have your adult partner write down) one thing you learned by completing the activity.

★ Place the Brave Point in your supercool Brave Points Bank.

ACTIVITY
18

Scary Pie Bake-Off

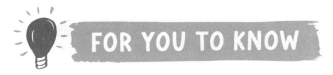

FOR YOU TO KNOW

Imagine you just entered a competition to see who can make the best pie. But this is no ordinary pie bake-off...this is a Scary Pie bake-off. A Scary Pie is a mixture of all the fears and worries that come together to make you feel super-duper anxious and uncomfortable.

Everyone's Scary Pie is unique to them. For example, some people like going to parties, while other people are terrified of being in a big group of people. Some people love going to the beach, while others think the idea of getting all sandy or swimming in the ocean to be awful.

What ingredients would you include to make your very own award-winning Scary Pie?

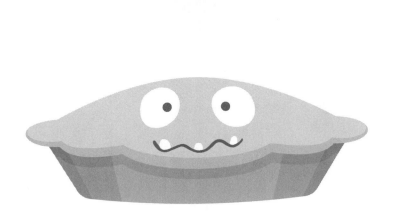

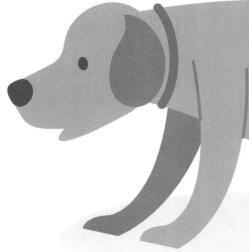

FOR YOU TO DO ⭐

STEP 1   Review the list below of the most common ingredients children have in their Scary Pies. For each ingredient, give a fear rating of 0 to 10, depending on how afraid you feel of this Scary Pie ingredient, with 0 being "it does not bother me at all" to 10 being "it terrifies me."

INGREDIENT FEAR RATING

SCARY PIE INGREDIENT	FEAR RATING (0–10)
The dark	
Going to the bathroom	
Thunder, lightning, and storms	
People wearing masks or costumes	
Sleeping alone	
Loud noises	
Talking to new people	
Getting in trouble at school	

Making a mistake	
Getting lost	
Water, beaches, or pools	
Being separated from your parents	
Doctors or dentists	
Bugs, insects, or animals	
Monsters	
Kids making fun of you	
Doing something embarrassing	
Being alone	
Getting sick or hurt	
Throwing up	
Something bad happening to parent(s)	
Other fear:	
Other fear:	
Other fear:	

STEP 2 Create your very own Scary Pie recipe card.

    1. List YOUR top 10 Scary Pie ingredients.

    2. List your current fear rating for each of them.

MY SCARY PIE RECIPE

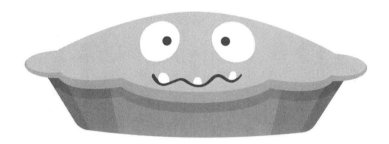

Date _____

	INGREDIENT	FEAR RATING		INGREDIENT	FEAR RATING
1.			6.		
2.			7.		
3.			8.		
4.			9.		
5.			10.		

☀ FOR YOU TO DISCUSS

Take turns answering these questions with your adult partner. After hearing each other's responses, take a moment to compliment each other for bravely discussing this important topic.

- What 10 ingredients you would put in your very own Scary Pie? How would you rate, on a 0 to 10 scale, just how scary each of these ingredients are?

- What ingredients would you have put in a Scary Pie when you were my age?

- Why do you think the ingredients of your Scary Pie today are different now? What has changed and why?

By completing this activity, you have earned a

Great job!

★ **Take a Brave Point from the storage bag.**

★ **On the back of the Brave Point, write down (or have your adult partner write down) one thing you learned by completing the activity.**

★ **Place the Brave Point in your supercool Brave Points Bank.**

From "Wow" to "Whatever"

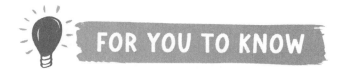

FOR YOU TO KNOW

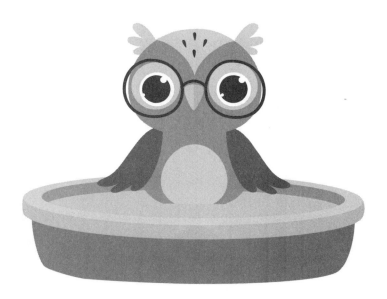

When you jump into a cold pool, at first your body feels the shock of the freezing water, and it takes your breath away. But after a little time, your body starts to get used to the water's temperature, and you begin to feel comfortable and enjoy the splish-splashing fun.

POP QUIZ Circle the best explanation you can think of as to why you start to feel less cold and more comfortable in a pool a few moments after you jump into it.

A. The water is getting warmer.

B. You are getting more used to the cold water.

If you selected B, you are correct! The water does not get warmer, but your body gets used to the pool's (at first chilly) temperature.

Guess what? You can get used to your fears and worries just like you get used to the cold water in a pool. Let's say you're scared of sleeping with the lights off. The first night you try it, you might feel a little jittery and afraid. You might hide under the covers more than usual, worried about the spooky things that could be lurking in the dark. You may think, *Wow, I'll never fall asleep!* But eventually, you will fall asleep.

The next night, you might still feel a bit nervous as you get into bed and your eyes adjust to the dark. But over time, you'll get used to sleeping in a cozy, dark room. You might even forget what it was like to want a bright night-light when you go to bed and simply think, *It's whatever, no big deal!* Just like your body gets used to the cold water of a pool, the same goes for your guard dog growing more comfortable with your Scary Pie ingredients.

FOR YOU TO DO ★

Don't just take our word for it! You deserve to witness for yourself the magic of your brain and body turning a "wow" into a "whatever."

ICY COLD TRANSFORMATION

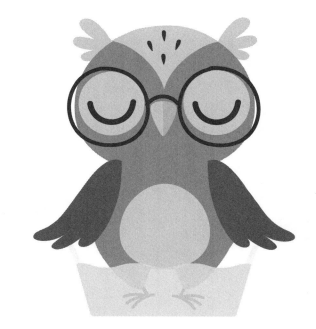

1. Have your adult partner fill a bathtub a few inches deep with cold water.

2. Step your bare feet into the cold bath.

3. How cold do your feet feel the first moment you put them in the water? (0 is not cold at all and 10 extremely cold)

4. After 10 seconds, how cold do your feet feel? (0–10)

5. After 20 seconds, how cold do your feet feel? (0–10)

6. After 30 seconds, how cold do your feet feel? (0–10)

SCENT ERASER

1. Have your adult partner pick a nice-smelling lotion.

2. Put a small amount of the yummy-smelling lotion on your hand.

3. Right after you put a bit on, smell your hand. How strong is the yummy smell? (0 is not strong smelling at all and 10 is extremely strong smelling)

4. Keep your nose on your hand and continue to smell the lotion.

5. After 10 seconds, how strong is the smell? (0–10)

6. After 20 seconds, how strong is the smell? (0–10)

7. After 30 seconds, how strong is the smell? (0–10)

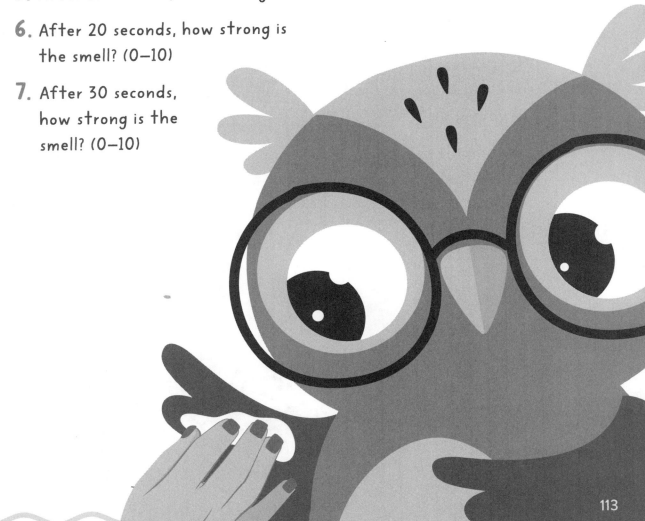

FROM POKEY TO OKEY-DOKEY

1. On a small piece of paper, write down one of your Scary Pie ingredients.

2. Crumple the piece of paper into a teeny tiny ball.

3. Place the paper in your shoe.

4. Notice what it feels like to have the pokey feeling in your shoe.

5. Right after you put the paper in your shoe, how pokey is the feeling? (0 is not at all pokey and 10 is extremely pokey)

6. Next, walk around for one minute. How pokey does the paper feel in your shoe? (0–10)

7. Next do 10 jumping jacks and then notice how pokey the paper feels in your shoe. (0–10)

8. Next find a ball and play one minute of catch with your adult partner and then notice how pokey the paper feels in your shoe. (0–10)

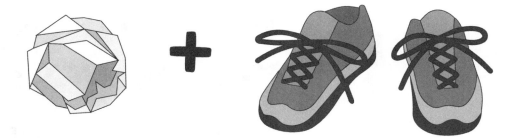

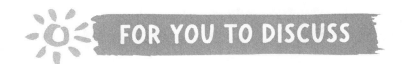

FOR YOU TO DISCUSS

Discuss your answers to the following questions with your adult partner:

- When you first tried these tests, how much did you notice the change? How sure were you that you would get used to them?

- After some time doing each test, what did you notice? What were you paying attention to?

- If you can get used to these tests, what else could you get used to?

By completing this activity, you have earned a

Great job!

★ Take a Brave Point from the storage bag.

★ On the back of the Brave Point, write down (or have your adult partner write down) one thing you learned by completing the activity.

★ Place the Brave Point in your supercool Brave Points Bank.

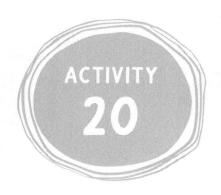

Fear Transformer

Like we talked about in the last activity, your brain and body are amazing at getting used to all kinds of things, including stuff that makes you feel scared. When you bravely face your fears, it's like showing your guard dog that everything's okay and there's no need to worry. It's similar to taking your guard dog around your house, showing it that everything is safe and there's no danger it needs to protect you from. That way, it can finally relax and be quiet.

FOR YOU TO DO

1. Write your top 10 Scary Pie ingredients at the top of each box on the next page.

2. For each Scary Pie ingredient, write down your current fear rating. (0 is not at all scary and 10 is extremely scary).

3. For each Scary Pie ingredient, write down the first five words that come to mind when you think of the fear.

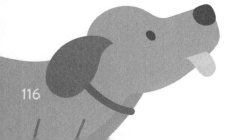

Ingredient 1

Initial Fear Rating:

1.
2.
3.
4.
5.

Ingredient 2

Initial Fear Rating:

1.
2.
3.
4.
5.

Ingredient 3

Initial Fear Rating:

1.
2.
3.
4.
5.

Ingredient 4

Initial Fear Rating:

1.
2.
3.
4.
5.

Ingredient 5

Initial Fear Rating:

1.
2.
3.
4.
5.

Ingredient 6

Initial Fear Rating:

1.
2.
3.
4.
5.

Ingredient 7

Initial Fear Rating:

1.
2.
3.
4.
5.

Ingredient 8

Initial Fear Rating:

1.
2.
3.
4.
5.

Ingredient 9

Initial Fear Rating:

1.
2.
3.
4.
5.

Ingredient 10

Initial Fear Rating:

1.
2.
3.
4.
5.

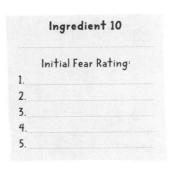

4. In the boxes below, draw a picture of each Scary Pie ingredient.

5. Take a second to again notice and write down your fear rating for each ingredient.

Ingredient 1

Fear Rating After
Facing Fear:

Ingredient 2

Fear Rating After
Facing Fear:

Ingredient 3

Fear Rating After
Facing Fear:

Ingredient 4

Fear Rating After
Facing Fear:

Ingredient 5

Fear Rating After
Facing Fear:

Ingredient 6

Fear Rating After
Facing Fear:

Ingredient 7

Fear Rating After
Facing Fear:

Ingredient 8

Fear Rating After
Facing Fear:

Ingredient 9

Fear Rating After
Facing Fear:

Ingredient 10

Fear Rating After
Facing Fear:

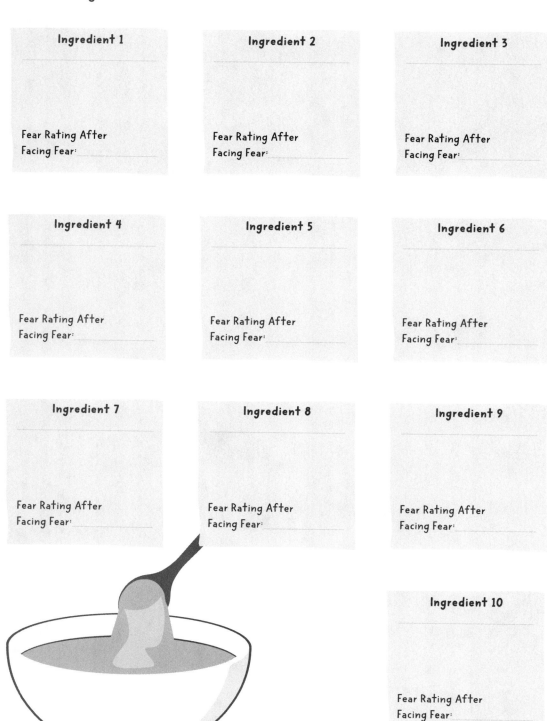

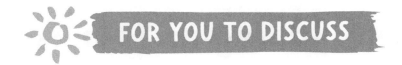
Discuss your answers to the following questions with your adult partner:

- Have any of your fear ratings changed after "jumping in the pool" and hanging out with these fears for a bit?

- Can you think of anything that you were scared of when you were little that now you are no longer afraid of?

- What do you think helped you to outgrow these fears?

By completing this activity, you have earned a

Great job!

★ Take a Brave Point from the storage bag.

★ On the back of the Brave Point, write down (or have your adult partner write down) one thing you learned by completing the activity.

★ Place the Brave Point in your supercool Brave Points Bank.

ACTIVITY
21

Rolling in Your Fears

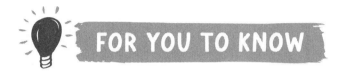

FOR YOU TO KNOW

Just like how you may start getting bored with even the most interesting toy after playing with it for a while, the same is true of your guard dog playing with your fears. The more time your guard dog spends hanging out with your fears, the calmer it will feel.

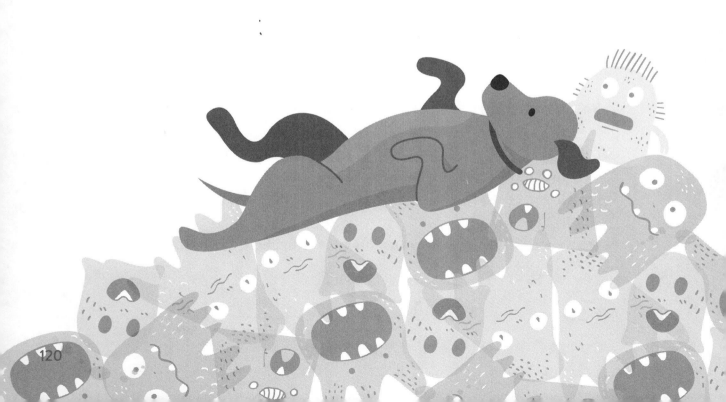

FOR YOU TO DO ☆

1. Gather supplies: 20 sticky notes of all shapes and sizes — the bigger the better! 10 are for you, and 10 are for your adult partner.

2. You and your adult partner both draw pictures or words related to the top 10 Scary Pie ingredients. Your adult partner will use their own top 10 Scary Pie ingredients.

3. Place each of your sticky notes with sticky-side up on the ground like the diagram below:

4. Count down from five, and together with your adult partner, roll on the ground. When you get up, count how many Scary Pie ingredients you've got sticking to you and which fears they are.

5. Whoever has the most Scary Pie ingredients stuck to them is the winner!!

☀️ FOR YOU TO DISCUSS

Take turns answering these questions with your adult partner. After hearing each other's responses, take a moment to compliment each other for bravely discussing this important topic.

● How does it feel to have your fears sticking to you?

● Are you surprised how much fun it can be to roll around in your fears?

By completing this activity, you have earned a

Great job!

★ Take a Brave Point from the storage bag.

★ On the back of the Brave Point, write down (or have your adult partner write down) one thing you learned by completing the activity.

★ Place the Brave Point in your supercool Brave Points Bank.

ACTIVITY 22

Scary Land

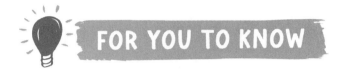

FOR YOU TO KNOW

Welcome to Scary Land, a game of fear busting challenges! To reach the Kingdom of the Brave, you will need to explore the Worry Woods, climb Panic Peak, and hunt for Scary Pie ingredients on Anxiety Island.

Along the way, you will complete brave steps from your Scary Pie ingredients list.

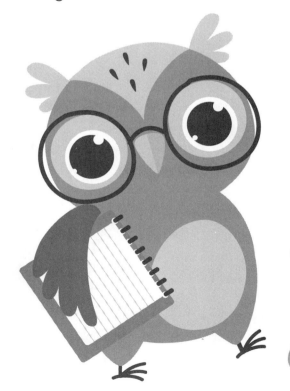

FOR YOU TO DO

The winner of this game is the person who arrives at the Kingdom of the Brave LAST. Yes, you read that correctly. To win Scary Land, you want to complete as many brave challenges as possible. Therefore, the longer it takes you to reach the finish line, the more practice you have playing with versus running from your Scary Pie ingredients.

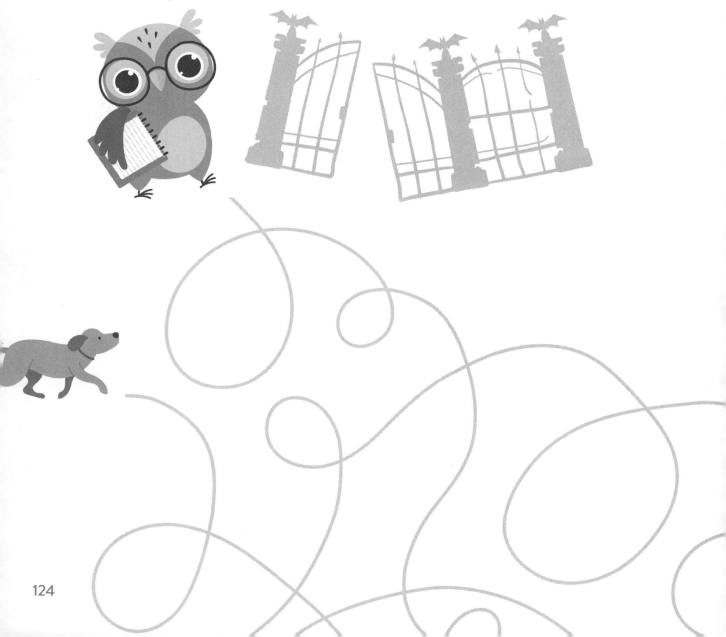

1. Gather supplies: 1 die, a piece of paper, and a pen or pencil.

2. Create a small character piece by drawing a "before" picture of yourself feeling scared and worried. On the other side of the piece of paper, draw an "after" picture of yourself feeling confident and brave.

3. Place your character pieces at the START box on the game board.

4. Since you and your adult partner are just beginning your journey to the Kingdom of the Brave, place your character pieces with the scared (before) picture facing up.

5. Roll the die and move your character piece the number of spaces listed on the die.

6. Complete the brave step listed on the game board as described.

7. Continue to roll the die and complete the brave steps until you both arrive at the Kingdom of the Brave.

8. Once you make it to the FINISH line, make sure to turn over your character piece to show the picture of the brave, confident you taking a victory lap.

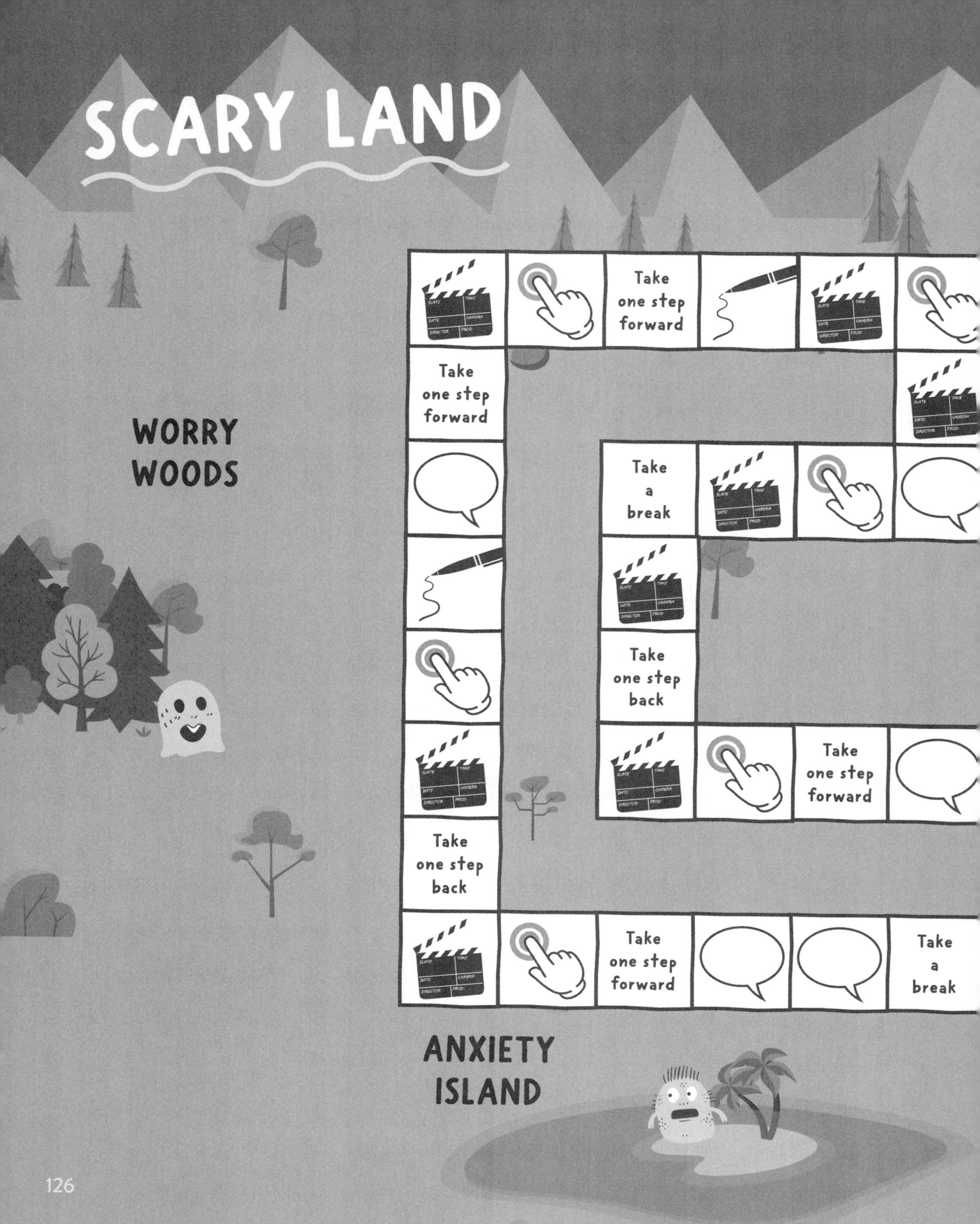

SCARY LAND

WORRY
WOODS

Take one step forward

Take one step forward

Take a break

Take one step back

Take one step forward

Take one step back

Take one step forward

Take a break

ANXIETY
ISLAND

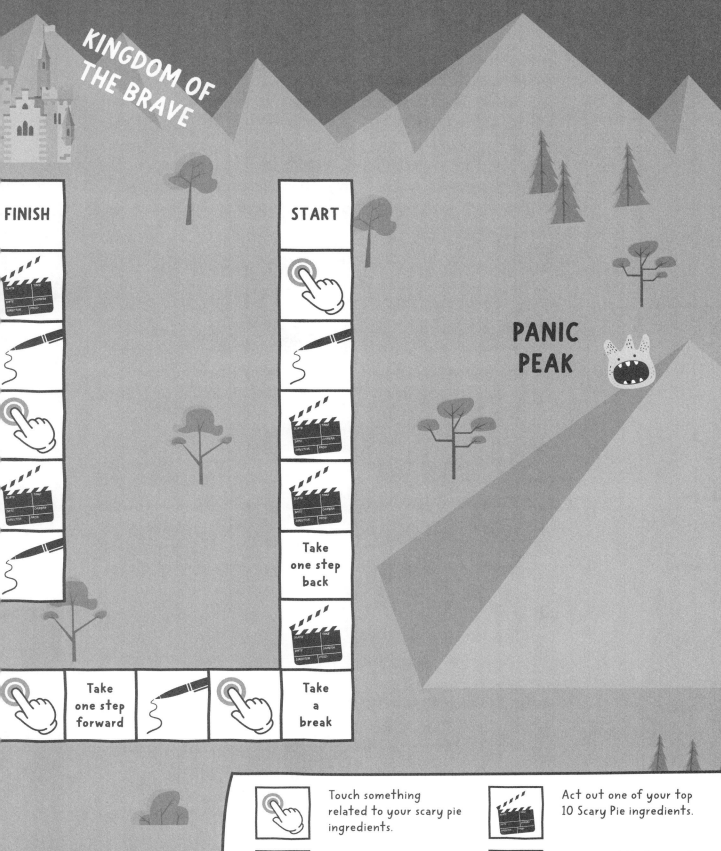

KINGDOM OF THE BRAVE

FINISH

START

PANIC PEAK

Take one step back

Take one step forward

Take a break

 Touch something related to your scary pie ingredients.

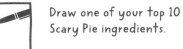 Act out one of your top 10 Scary Pie ingredients.

Draw one of your top 10 Scary Pie ingredients.

 Say a word that reminds you of your top 10 Scary Pie ingredients.

Take turns answering these questions with your adult partner. After hearing each other's responses, take a moment to compliment each other for bravely discussing this important topic.

- What was it like to take the brave steps during the game? How loud did your guard dog bark at you during these challenges?

- Was the Scary Land Game as difficult to play as you thought it would be?

- What do you think would happen if you played the game again? Would your guard dog bark as much and just as loudly? Or would it feel calmer after playing with the same Scary Pie ingredients?

By completing this activity, you have earned a

Great job!

★ Take a Brave Point from the storage bag.

★ On the back of the Brave Point, write down (or have your adult partner write down) one thing you learned by completing the activity.

★ Place the Brave Point in your supercool Brave Points Bank.

ACTIVITY 23

The Get It Wrong Game

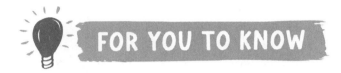

FOR YOU TO KNOW

Your guard dog is like your very own built-in "mistake checker." It's always on the lookout, reviewing what you are doing to make sure you don't mess up or do anything wrong. It's worried that if you make a mistake, something really bad might happen, like getting into trouble or having people not like you.

But all of this mistake-checking work is exhausting for your guard dog and for you. And the kicker is, all this hard work is for nothing. No matter how hard your guard dog works and no matter how much you listen to it and do everything in your power to make sure you never ever make a mistake, it is impossible for any of us humans to be perfect.

But say it would be possible to live a perfectly perfect life (which it is not), this would be a super boring way to exist. It would be like living in a beautiful, quiet museum where nothing ever changes. There would be no adventures, no trying new things, and no interesting exploring to do. That doesn't sound like a fun way to live, does it?

The good news is that life is full of chances to make healthy mistakes. Every time you make a mistake, it means you're being brave and trying something new. But your guard dog may need some extra training to learn how helpful and actually fun it can be to get things wrong and live a perfectly imperfect life.

FOR YOU TO DO ⭐

In order to teach your guard dog how to live a perfectly imperfect life, you and your adult partner are going to play the Get It Wrong Game. In this exercise, you two are going to have a ton of fun getting things wrong!

1. Review with your adult partner the first 12 examples of Get It Wrong challenges.

2. Together, come up with 4 additional Get It Wrong challenges and fill in the last row of the Get It Wrong Game sheet.

3. Now you are ready to play the Get It Wrong Game!

   - Take turns selecting a Get It Wrong challenge by closing your eyes and then putting your finger down anywhere on the game sheet.

   - Do the Get It Wrong challenge and try to really mess it up as much as possible!

   - If your finger lands somewhere on the sheet that does not have a challenge, such as the blank area on the side of the page, go you! You win bonus points for getting it wrong even before you did your actual challenge. Just close your eyes and randomly pick another spot on the page and keep going until you land on or close to a challenge.

   - Try to play at least 5 rounds of the Get It Wrong Game, so you and your adult partner each have plenty of chances to delight in how silly and freeing it feels to embrace making mistakes.

THE GET IT WRONG GAME

Create a strange snack combination, like peanut butter and pickles, and taste-test them with your partner.

Walk around the room in silly ways, like hopping like a bunny or waddling like a penguin.

Put on the wackiest outfit possible by mixing and matching clothes in unexpected ways.

Create an obstacle course using pillows and blankets. Now move through it and bump into as many things as possible.

Tell an unfunny, corny joke.

Ask your partner a question in a made-up language they can't understand.

Tell a really boring story to your partner.

Draw a portrait of your partner with your eyes closed. Sign your MESSterpiece.

Your partner draws a picture and tells you "color carefully." Now close your eyes and color!

Have a slow race against your partner. The winner is the person who gets to the finish line LAST.

Answer this math problem WRONG:

$1+1=?$

Take a sip of water and "by accident" spill some water on your shirt.

Make up your own Get It Wrong challenge.

Make up your own Get It Wrong challenge.

Make up your own Get It Wrong challenge.

Make up your own Get It Wrong challenge.

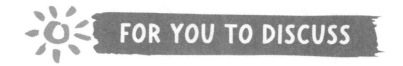

FOR YOU TO DISCUSS

Take turns answering these questions with your adult partner. After hearing each other's responses, take a moment to compliment each other for bravely discussing this important topic.

- What do you think is good about playing the Get It Wrong Game?

- How comfortable do you feel getting things wrong?

- Is getting things wrong a skill that you think is important for you to continue to work on?

- Do you wish someone had played the Get It Wrong Game with you and showed you how fun it can be to get things wrong, when you were my age?

- How can you continue to find creative ways to practice getting things wrong each and every day, for the rest of our lives?

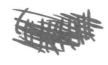

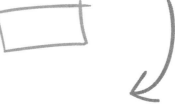

By completing this activity, you have earned a

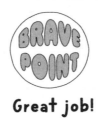

Great job!

★ Take a Brave Point from the storage bag.

★ On the back of the Brave Point, write down (or have your adult partner write down) one thing you learned by completing the activity.

★ Place the Brave Point in your supercool Brave Points Bank.

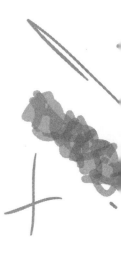

ACTIVITY 24

Best in Show

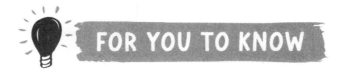

It's time for a special event with your guard dog! You and your guard dog are invited to the Best-Trained Guard Dog Show.

The Best-Trained Guard Dog Show is like a talent show for guard dogs. Here, your guard dog can showcase all its amazing tricks and impress everyone with its bravery and skills. Your guard dog has been working really hard to learn how to bark less and stay calm, and now it's time to show off these cool new tricks it has learned.

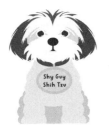

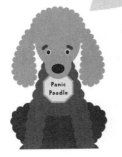

CALLING ALL GUARD DOGS

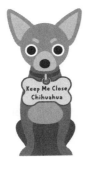

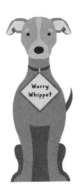

You and your guard dog are invited to an unforgettable day of brave tricks and fun!

Best-Trained Guard Dog Show is your guard dog's chance to show off just how well trained and brave it can be!

Sign up now to secure your spot on stage!

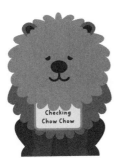

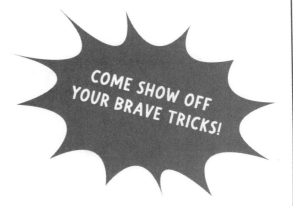

COME SHOW OFF YOUR BRAVE TRICKS!

The key to a successful talent show is to pick which talent you want to show off.

See the list below of the most common tricks that are challenging and awe-inspiring for each guard dog type. The most impressive brave tricks are going to depend on the guard dog. For example, sleeping in its own room might not be a big deal for the Worry Whippet. However, going on a trip without knowing all the details of the plan is more impressive because this dog worries more about what's going to happen next than monsters under the bed. For the Keep Me Close Chihuahua, going with the flow on a trip and not knowing the plan may not be a big deal, but sleeping alone throughout the night would call for a standing ovation from the adoring crowd.

Your goal is to pick five supercool brave tricks from the following list. These tricks will wow everyone with just how awesome and well trained your guard dog has become! Choose tricks that are not too easy or too tough—just the right amount of challenge to make your guard dog a superstar.

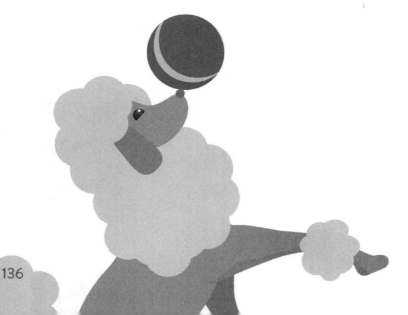

GUARD DOG TRICKS

SHY GUY SHIH TSU	KEEP ME CLOSE CHIHUAHUA	PANIC POODLE	WORRY WHIPPET	CHECKING CHOW CHOW
Say hi to someone you don't know very well.	Spend time alone in a room, with the door shut, as far away from the room your parents are in as possible.	Spend a few minutes in a crowded, loud space (with your adult partner).	Make a small mistake on purpose.	Go to bed without checking to make sure doors are locked.
Say something silly to a friend.	Have a sleepover at a friend's or family member's house.	Spend time in an unfamiliar environment, without knowing when you will be leaving.	Draw a picture of something that could go wrong in the future.	Touch something germy.
Speak your own order to a waiter at a restaurant.	Sleep in your own room for the whole night.	Breathe fast, spin around, and make your body feel as panicky and weird as possible!	Be a few minutes late to something.	Don't text or call your parents when they are out.
Make Up Your Own Brave Trick	Make Up Your Own Brave Trick	Make Up Your Own Brave Trick	Make Up Your Own Brave Trick	Make Up Your Own Brave Trick

Each time you complete a trick, color in a section of the award ribbon below. Once you have done five tricks, your guard dog has won best in show!

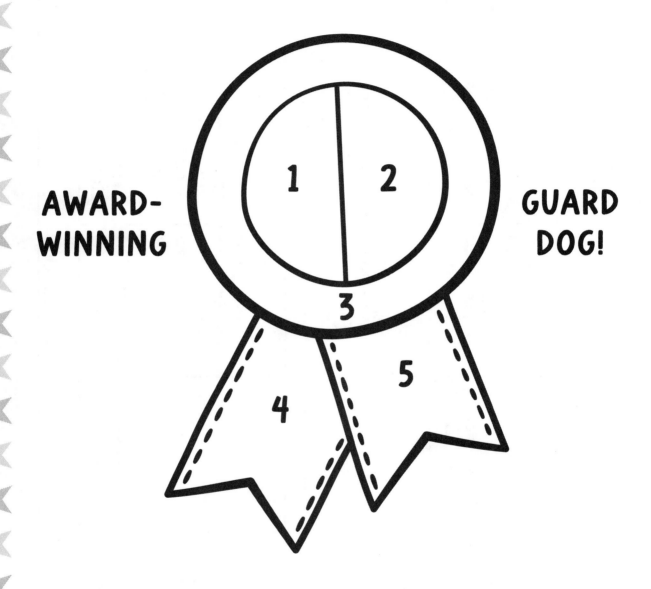

AWARD-
WINNING

GUARD
DOG!

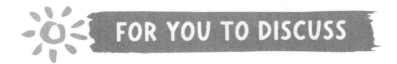

FOR YOU TO DISCUSS

Discuss your answers to the following questions with your adult partner:

- How hard was it for your guard dog to perform these tricks?

- Were some tricks harder to perform than others?

- What did it feel like to color in the fifth section of ribbon after doing the final trick? We hope you felt proud of yourself and your well-trained guard dog!

By completing this activity, you have earned a

Great job!

★ Take a Brave Point from the storage bag.

★ On the back of the Brave Point, write down (or have your adult partner write down) one thing you learned by completing the activity.

★ Place the Brave Point in your supercool Brave Points Bank.

ACTIVITY 25

BraveWare

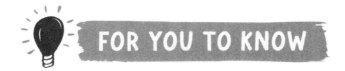

FOR YOU TO KNOW

There will be times when your guard dog barks really loudly, and it might be tough to remember all the wonderful lessons you've learned in this brave adventure book. That's why it's helpful to keep these lessons handy, so you can use them when you need them most—like when you're about to give up something important just to stop feeling scared.

We've had the chance to learn from our amazing and brave friends, and they have given us some cool tips and reminders to share about working their brave muscles and doing important things, even when it's hard and scary.

Here are some of the top helpful reminders we've learned:

★   Just because my guard dog is barking "DANGER!" doesn't mean it's true.

★   If I keep going, the scary feelings will soon pass.

★   I can teach my guard dog that it's safe to relax.

★   I may not like feeling scared, but I can handle it.

★   To do the fun things I want to do, I might have to feel scared sometimes.

But here's the thing: what works for one person might not work for another. That's why it's important to come up with a few "brave reminders" that work best for YOU.

You're the expert on you, and you know what will be most helpful when you face those tricky moments. You've done such great work during this brave journey. What has helped you face your fears? What do you remind yourself of to take that next step, even when you feel scared and uncomfortable?

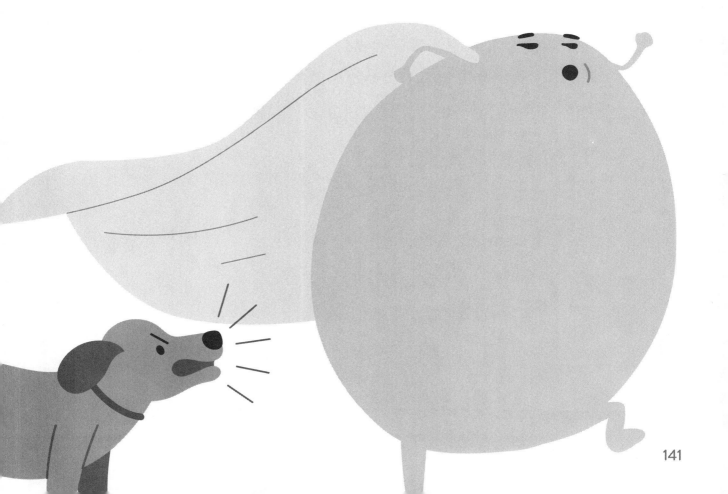

FOR YOU TO DO ⭐

Think about one of the brave challenges you have done recently. What did you tell yourself to push forward, to tolerate the short-term discomfort to get the immediate reward of the Brave Point and the longer-term reward of a bigger and better life?

Draw a picture of the first thing that comes to mind when you think about being brave and doing something that is important to you, even when your guard dog is experiencing a false alarm and barking danger at you.

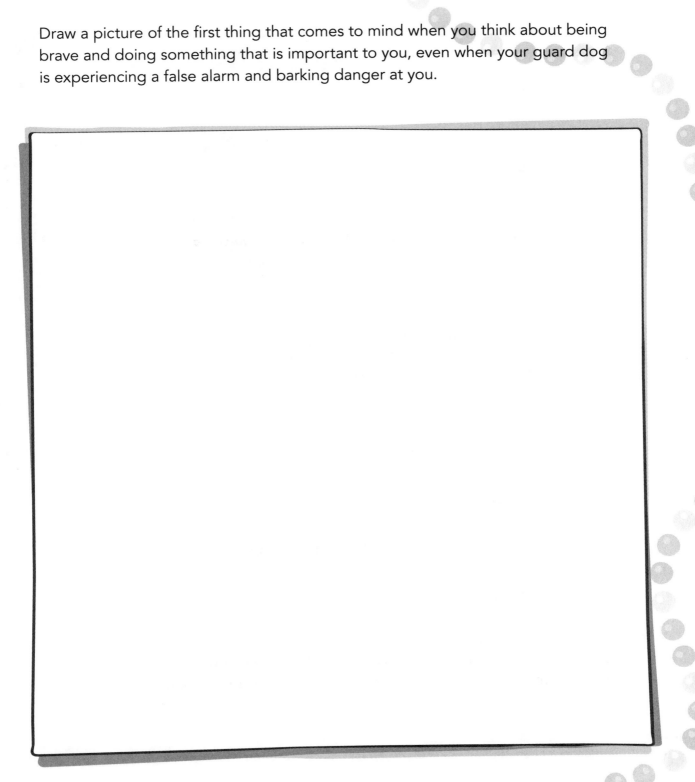

In order to take this reminder "on the road" with you, so you can have it when you need it most, you are going to design your very own BraveWare jewelry line.

Your jewelry line:

1. Think of a few words or images that come to mind when you think about being brave.

   Your brave reminder does not have to be a whole sentence. It does not have to be perfect. It just has to give you a quick boost of extra fuel to help you keep going and face your fear when your guard dog is stuck in false-alarm mode.

2. Sketch out a few ideas for your BraveWare jewelry line.

3. Have your adult partner take you to an art store and buy some supplies to create your BraveWare jewelry.

   Sample supplies to purchase:

   - Letter beads

   - Beads with graphics or images that inspire you

   - String or elastic cord

See a few fantastic examples on the next page made by our brave friends, who wowed us with their creativity and determination to live their best life:

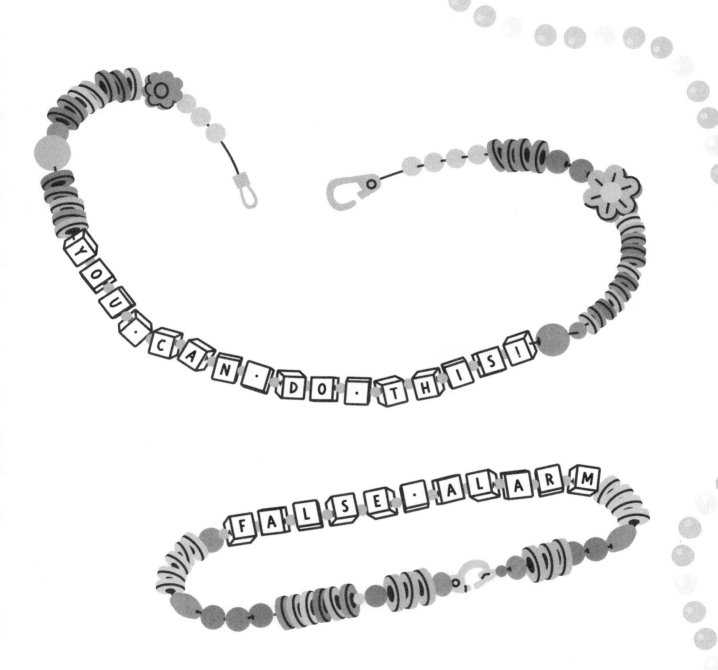

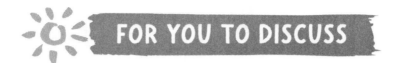

Ask your adult partner:

- What do you tell yourself to coach yourself forward in order to do hard but important things?

- What would you put on your own BraveWare jewelry piece? (Surprise them and make one for them!)

Discuss how your adult partner can help you when your guard dog is barking at you and you're stuck in your fears and worries.

- What do you want them to say to you?

- What would you like them to do?

- What do you NOT want them to say or do?

By completing this activity, you have earned a

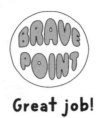

Great job!

★ Take a Brave Point from the storage bag.

★ On the back of the Brave Point, write down (or have your adult partner write down) one thing you learned by completing the activity.

★ Place the Brave Point in your supercool Brave Points Bank.

Celebration Station!

It's time to use your Brave Points to get your fantastic prizes!

- Get your Brave Point Bank, take out your 25 Brave Points, and give them to your adult partner.

- Discuss with your adult partner when and how you'll exchange your points for the prizes you wanted.

- You can also chat together and see if you've discovered new interests and exciting prizes that you'd love. Your grown-up partner can help you decide on changing prizes if you have some new favorites.

Besides these awesome prizes, you've also won something even more super special: a bigger and more exciting life! You've learned the secret of taming your anxiety guard dog and tuning in to the helpful advice of your wise owl.

Although you've reached the end of this book, your brave adventure continues! Just like brushing your teeth every day for a healthy smile, you also need to exercise your "brave muscles" daily for a healthy life. By facing, rather than avoiding, things that make you scared and stressed a little bit every day, you'll keep your life big and exciting, and your guard dog will stay tame and calm.

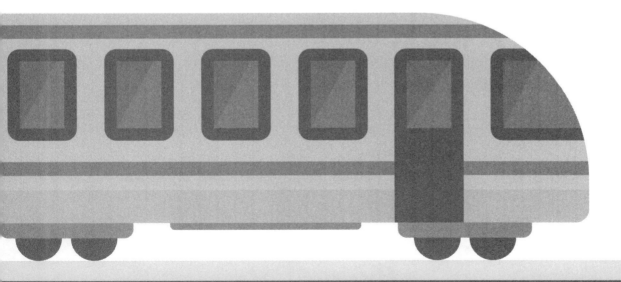

Debra Kissen, PhD, is a clinical psychologist, and CEO of the Light On Anxiety Treatment Centers. She is author of several books on cognitive behavioral therapy (CBT)-focused management of anxiety, worry, panic, and fear, including *The Panic Workbook for Teens*, *Rewire Your Anxious Brain for Teens*, and *Break Free from Intrusive Thoughts*.

Meena Dugatkin, PsyD, is a licensed clinical child psychologist at Light On Anxiety Treatment Centers. She specializes in evidence-based CBT and exposure and response prevention (ERP) treatments to help children and teens struggling with anxiety and obsessive-compulsive disorder (OCD).

Grace Cusack, LPC, works with families and clients of all ages at Light On Anxiety Treatment Centers, has advanced training in ERP and CBT, and helps her clients develop symptom awareness and coping strategies for anxiety, OCD, and other related disorders.

MORE BOOKS from
NEW HARBINGER PUBLICATIONS

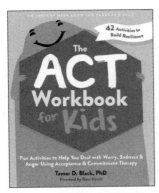
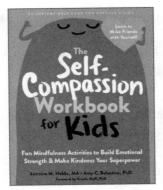
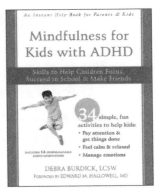
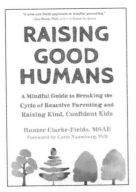
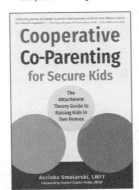
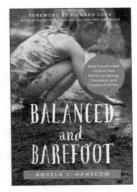

Did you know there are **free tools** you can download for this book?

Free tools are things like **worksheets, guided meditation exercises**, and **more** that will help you get the most out of your book.

You can download free tools for this book— whether you bought or borrowed it, in any format, from any source—from the New Harbinger website. All you need is a NewHarbinger.com account. Just use the URL provided in this book to view the free tools that are available for it. Then, click on the "download" button for the free tool you want, and follow the prompts that appear to log in to your NewHarbinger.com account and download the material.

You can also save the free tools for this book to your **Free Tools Library** so you can access them again anytime, just by logging in to your account! Just look for this button on the book's free tools page.

+ Save this to my free tools library

If you need help accessing or downloading free tools, visit **newharbinger.com/faq** or contact us at **customerservice@newharbinger.com**.